I0414448

OBESITY

A COMPREHENSIVE REVIEW

THE WHO, WHAT, WHEN, WHY, WHERE AND HOW OF THE OBESITY PROBLEM

E. PATRICK ALLEYNE

D.I.C.T.A, M.SC, M.S.A, PH.D

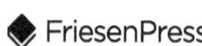 FriesenPress

One Printers Way
Altona, MB R0G 0B0
Canada

www.friesenpress.com

ISBN
978-1-03-918800-6 (Hardcover)
978-1-03-918799-3 (Paperback)
978-1-03-918801-3 (eBook)

1. HEALTH & FITNESS, WEIGHT LOSS

Distributed to the trade by The Ingram Book Company

Dedication

I dedicate this review to my children: Patricia, Allyson-Dale, Susannah, and Andrew. Individually unique, each one a tremendous source of joy and inspiration throughout my life's journey.

ACKNOWLEDGEMENTS

THE COMPLETION OF this project, whatever the concluding judgement, was enabled by significant voluntary contributions and sustained inspirational encouragement from many sources. Professor Allan Johnson remains the stalwart in guiding me with respect to critical content. My dear friend and colleague, Dr. Lystra Fletcher-Paul provided considerable sustained inspiration and kept me going. She emphasised no-nonsense correction of style in early drafts. The venerable Dr. Chelston Brathwaite blessed me with a rude awakening of the task ahead and facilitated some critical thinking. Bruce Lauckner allowed me to benefit from his cumulative experience in the world of science editing and stayed the. length of the journey in the evolution of the manuscript.

The tremendous skill and patience of Jeneill Harris in the final days of getting the manuscript ready was a blessing in completing the exercise.

Good friends: Steve, Jennifer, and Ingrid kept me afloat on inspirational whispers throughout the voyage. To all of you, I am eternally grateful.

Table of Contents

Introduction 1

1. Fat 5

2. Breakfast: How Important Is This Meal? 21

3. Water: Discover the Miracle of Nature. 27

4. Digestion: The Search for Energy—Carbohydrates,
    Starches, Sugars, and Proteins. 40

5. Digestive Enzymes and Gastrointestinal Health:
    Intolerance, Resistance, Sensitivity, and MCTs. 56

6. Selected Prominent Diet Types as Systems
    of Aggressive Food-Intake Control. 71

7. Gut Bacteria: The Microbiome 93

8. Plant-Based Whole Foods and Calorie Density:
    Elements of Control for Effective Dietary Patterns 108

9. Exercise Part 1: Selected General Information 126

10. Exercise Part 2: Walking: A Popular Form of
    Exercise for All Ages. 154

11. Individual and Societal Costs: The Prevalence
    of Overweight and Obesity Issues. 163

12. Selected Tips: Managing Lifestyle Changes
    Considered Necessary for Combating Obesity. 174

References 191

Additional Recommended Resources. 203

Introduction

THE DECISION TO pursue a comprehensive review on this topic of personal health, and specifically the problem of excess weight management and obesity, arose in a very roundabout manner. I have been interested in the subject area for quite some time, for personal and family-related reasons, but more so as a topic of growing global concern with respect to the general "wellness" of society.

Obesity is now clearly regarded as a major global economic problem of "crisis" proportions. Estimates range considerably indicate from a low prevalence of 20%–30% and rising in some countries. In general, however, the rates are much higher. In North America, 70% of the population is overweight or obese; similar projections are seen for some other developed countries. The reported levels are increasingly alarming in developing countries.

The incidence of obesity, however, is reportedly highest in developing countries. The situation is exacerbated in "emerging economies" when there is a shift in social status as a result of an increase in average income and consequently wealth distribution. This change in social status is accompanied by dietary changes, especially an increased consumption of fast foods because of the change in lifestyles. These fast foods are often rich in salt, sugar, fats, and processed carbohydrates, all of which contribute to obesity. It is of interest to note that on September 1, 2023, a popular TV channel [CNN] announced that with respect to the global "weight-loss frenzy" the stock for Novo Nordisk in Denmark had achieved a value much bigger than the country itself.

Moreover, global expenditure to deal with obesity is estimated to be in the range of billions of dollars. Increasing resource allocation for research and education of the general population is very evident in both developed and developing countries

All this is taking place at the same time when food insecurity remains an area of major concern on a global basis:

Percentage Food Insecurity by Regions in 2021 (Littlemore, 2022)

	Moderate and Severe	Severe
N. America/Europe	8.0	1.5
Asia	24.6	10.5
Oceania	13.0	4.5
Africa	57.9	23.4
Latin America/Caribbean	40.6	14.2

Some one billion people are reported as being under-nourished and another two billion as malnourished. It is estimated that the world food supply will have to increase by 70% in 2050 in order to feed a global population of close to ten billion.

My broad-based scientific career exposed me to related research and development in the fields of agriculture, food production, and nutrition. This has been further enhanced by administrative and consulting responsibilities in various countries around the world. Based on these experiences, I have concluded that addressing this problem of obesity requires interventions at several levels by decision-makers, researchers, producers, and consumers of food. However, ultimately, the decision to change behaviour to enable an individual to achieve sustainable and appropriate weight management is a personal choice. This book, therefore, provides the reader with information to inform and assist in making the right choices.

My first inclination with this project was simply to produce a very short review of some of the essential elements related to obesity. However, an increasing level of excitement left me with a feeling to do more. I decided to research and prepare a comprehensive publication in simple language that the non-scientist could read and find interesting. In reality, I aimed at producing a document that most individuals, including students with broad-based academic exposure, would find both interesting and a useful source of information.

Each chapter is divided into subsections, which will enable the reader to decide, based on their interest, whether to read further within a chapter, depending on the details provided in the subsection. Feedback suggests some reasonable success in this regard. The reader is, therefore, guaranteed sufficient, valuable information to guide behaviour of the individual faced with carrying around more body fat than is considered medically acceptable and healthy.

Ravenous competition is evident in the search for sustainable measures to control obesity. Society cannot legislate corrective behaviour for individuals. In this regard, knowledge of the *why* and *what* takes place in the human body is crucial to effective weight management. An overview of the literature indicates that a host of individuals have been in search of special diets, magic formulas in the form of pills, potions, concoctions; even creams and exotic herbal infusions.

The media offers no end to products "proven" to manage obesity—some based on discoveries from far-away places and native peoples, some supposedly based on research by students in prestigious universities, and many of them representative of the explosive fraudulence which has emerged.

In this book, material is sought from a wide range of sources; an attempt is made to present findings from scientific literature in a simplified format. The reader can choose to take it all in or focus on areas of specific interest. Key concepts are emphasized along the way.

The material explains what takes place in the human body and *why* some changes in the way we live are necessary to achieve success with effective management of obesity. Three essentials emerge and are emphasised: what goes in, what comes out, and the need to move your body to expend energy.

Ultimately, there are no meaningful "shortcuts," and failure with one or more diets or exercise regimes can be disheartening. Rollercoaster experiences abound. Individual initiatives to combat obesity are loaded with wasted expenditure, high levels of failure, and abandoned human effort, at times ending in self-hate.

Success in the management of obesity is not an easy task. Patience and persistence will be tested. Believe ! It can be achieved. Whoever you may be; keep the faith; enjoy the journey.

May, 2024

CHAPTER 1
FAT

IN THE WORLD of nutrition, fat is one of the three macronutrients: carbohydrates, proteins, and fat. Carbohydrates and proteins are dealt with in some detail in later chapters of this book. Given that the word "fat" is an upfront reference in the overall context of this publication, I feel it necessary to ensure some minimum critical information be available on the particular subject area.

It is common to hear the term "fat molecule," also occasionally referred to as fatty acids or lipids. Other related terminology includes "lipocytes" and "fat cells". They are the cells that primarily compose adipose tissue; they specialise in storing energy as fat.

Molecules are formed when two or more atoms bind together. Atoms are the basic building blocks from which everything we know in existence is built. Fat molecules consist primarily of carbon and hydrogen. You will become familiar with some different types throughout this book. They are important substances of which one must be aware in the pursuit of ways of managing obesity at any level.

FATS ARE IMPORTANT

Fats are an important part of a healthy diet; they are a major source of fuel or energy, and they play important roles in the absorption of vitamins and the insulation of the body. For persons who are concerned about eating too much, fats help to give a feeling of fullness and can lead to reduced food intake.

Some foods have almost no fats, such as fruits and vegetables. Others have lots of fat; for example, nuts, oils, butter, and meats. It is, therefore, important to know which fats are regarded as healthy fats and to be aware of which fats abound in the major broad fatty food groupings.

Generally, unsaturated fats (both mono- and poly-) are the healthy group of fats and are found in plant foods, fish, and some oils. They are good for heart health and generally recommended in place of saturated fats and trans-fats. Sources containing "friendly" fats are salmon, avocados, olive, walnuts, and vegetable oils (soyabean, corn, canola, and olive oils).

On the matter of dietary intake, the important issues are the kinds and quantities of fat we consume, and the sources. Their relevance to human health is partially indicated by at least one estimate which projects global losses in human life each year of about fourteen million due to consumption of foods high in trans-fat, saturated fat, and sugar (Greger, 2019).

HOW IS FAT FORMED

In a later chapter, the term "calorie" is introduced. It represents a measure of energy used by the body to execute important metabolic processes related to the overall functioning of the body.

When we consume more calories (energy) than what is used up in metabolic processes and physical activity, the excess is stored as body fat. The storage takes place in specialised fat cells called adipose tissue. These storage cells may already exist and become enlarged, or additional fat-cell formation may take place.

Individuals vary in the extent to which they accumulate excess fat and gain weight based on their eating habits. Some remain thin; others struggle with problems of obesity. The difference is not accounted for only by consumption behaviour. It is recognised that inheritance elements (gene patterns) and the environment influence the final outcome. In essence, there are a few factors at play. The individual case story commences at birth and seems to hold throughout adult life. Recent modifications in scientific thought on this subject are mentioned later in the text

A simple explanation to keep in mind as it relates to the deposition of fat is that of how much you burn compared to how much you consume. If you want to avoid gaining weight, the former must exceed the latter. Reduced food consumption, such as reduced calorie intake, or burning more calories via exercise or other physical activity than you utilise for normal body functions leads to reduced fat storage, shrinking fat cells, and very likely a reduced waistline.

On matters relating to food consumption, we also learn that there are two major groups of fats: saturated and unsaturated, the latter being divided into three groups.

UNSATURATED FATS

Unsaturated fats include polyunsaturated, monounsaturated, and trans (trans-fatty acid) fats.

Trans-fats are associated with numerous negative health effects. It is found naturally in meat and dairy products, and is also created artificially when liquid vegetable oils are converted into semi-solid, partially hydrogenated oil by the addition of hydrogen. Trans-fats make up 3%–10% of the total fat in dairy products and meats, and is often added to processed foods to improve taste, texture, and longevity. It raises LDL-cholesterol (bad cholesterol) and lowers HDL-cholesterol (good cholesterol), and is considered the worse kind of fat one can eat since it increases the risk of heart disease.

Frequent sources of trans-fats include deep fried foods; ready-to-eat frozen foods; commercially baked goods, such as doughnuts; convenience foods; salty snack foods, such as popcorn, chips, and crackers; and packaged sweet snacks, such as cookies, cakes, and granola bars.

Food labels reading "hydrogenated" or "partially hydrogenated" oils are an indication of included trans-fats. Avoid them.

SATURATED FAT

Saturated fats contain a high proportion of fatty acid molecules with a simpler structural format. They are generally considered to be less healthy in the diet compared to unsaturated fat and are found in meat, other animal products, such as cheese and butter, and also in palm and coconut oils.

It is recommended that they be limited to a maximum of about 10% of one's diet in the daily choice of calories. Excessive consumption is associated with negative heart health conditions and high blood pressure.

WHO IS FAT? ARE YOU FAT?

Being "overfat" is having excess body fat sufficient to impair health. Any assessment, which results in an individual falling into this category, should be a wake-up call for immediate action to address the problem.

Usually, the focal point of reference in this situation becomes excess belly fat. An examination of North American data suggests about 71% of adults are overweight, as many as 90% are overfat, and between 33% and 40% of men and women have enough body fat to be classified as obese.

Indications are that mirrors do not lie. If you want to know if you are obese, try the mirror method; undress and look at yourself in the mirror.

Your Mirror Will Not Lie: Obesity Is Evident
[Drawings courtesy Kamau Paul, 2023l]

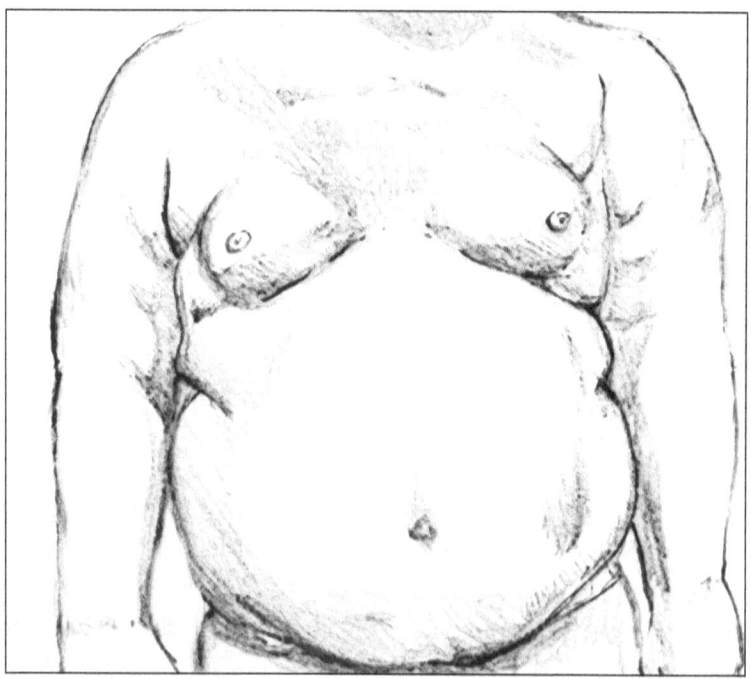

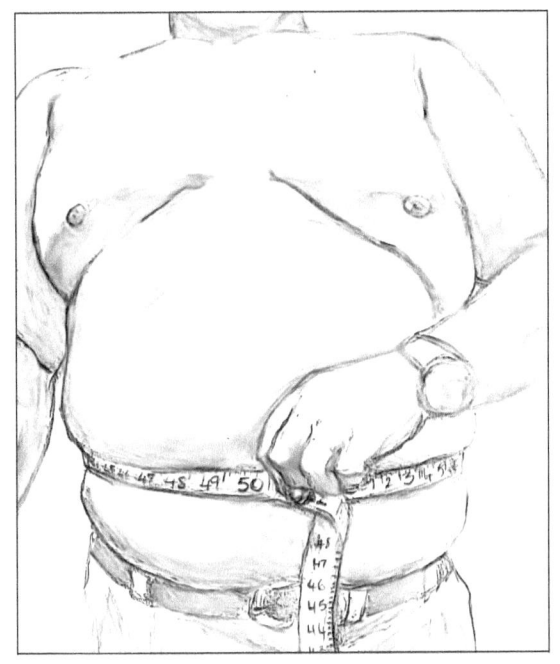

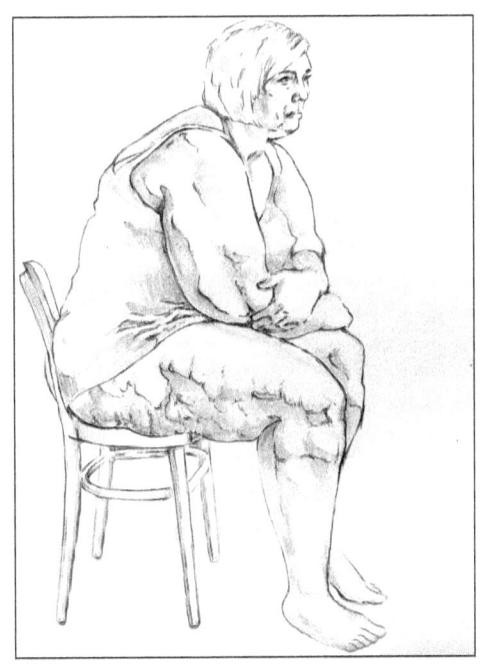

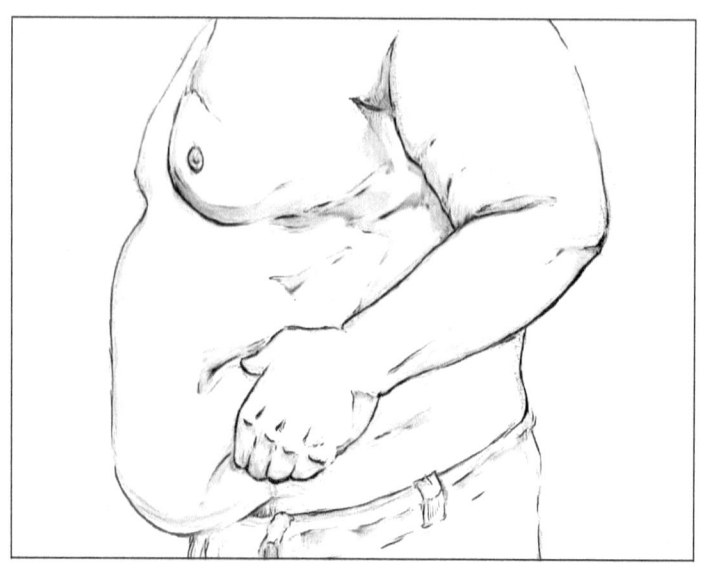

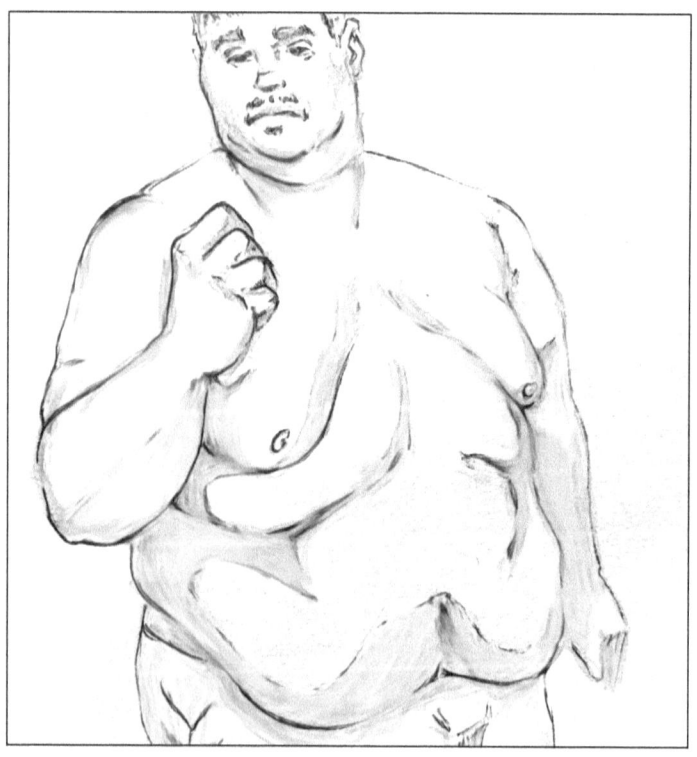

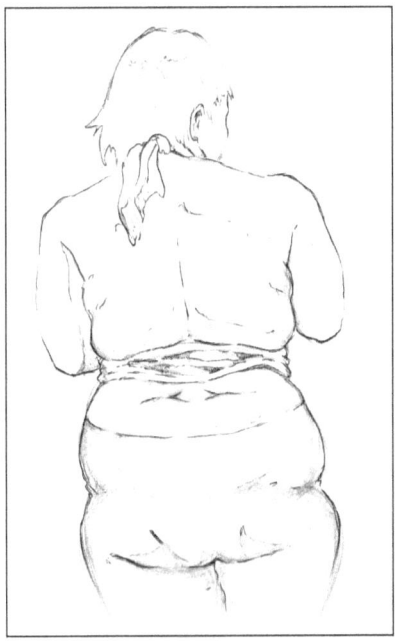

OBESITY: WHAT IS IT?

A simple definition of being overweight is <u>that</u> you have too much body fat. Whereas being obese, you have *way too much* body fat!

Obesity is defined, scientifically, as having a body mass index (BMI) of 30 kg/m² or more (Greger, 2019). Not everyone considers the matter in the same light. Fat activists apparently downplay the health risks of the condition and are involved in fighting size stigma, fat shaming, and discrimination. When we examine the possibility of what I choose to call the "positive double F" effect ("fat" and "fit"), the conclusion seems to be that it is just a matter of time before the risk factors develop. In due course, even "metabolically healthy," obese individuals are at an increased risk of diabetes, fatty liver disease, cardiovascular events such as heart attacks, and premature death.

The reference to healthy obesity seems to be a myth, but there may well be the possibility of a rare subgroup of obese individuals who do not suffer the typical metabolic costs of obesity, sometimes classified as "benign obesity."

Assessment of Body Fat (Percent Body Fat, BMI, and Waist Circumference)

Since obesity is defined as excess body fat, it should be assessed using the level of body fat (% of body fat); however, methods used for measurement of body fat are expensive and not suitable for large population sizes. Therefore, BMI is used as a proxy measure of body fat level.

BMI is based on height and weight. It can be calculated in either British or metric units using the formulae below:

$$\text{British units: } \mathbf{BMI} = (\text{weight } [\mathbf{lb}] \div \text{height}^2 \text{ [in.]}) \times 703$$
$$\text{Metric units: BMI} = \text{weight (kg)} \div \text{height}^2 \text{ (m)}$$

BMI, however, may underestimate the real prevalence of obesity since it does not consider the composition of the weight (fat, lean body mass [muscle], bone, and water) and the distribution of fat in the body of the individual. For example, an athlete or body builder with muscular builds could be classified as overweight or obese. Further, muscle tissue weighs more than fat tissue. Therefore, BMI measurement, by itself, may lead to misclassification of the individual.

The World Health Organization and the American College of Endocrinology define obesity as being over 25% in men and 35% in women. When applied to the American population in the 1990s, BMI measurements indicated a 20% obesity rate compared to about 50% using percentage fat. More importantly, BMI as an indicator is a better predictor of cardiovascular disease.

For general assessment purposes, BMI is classified in adults as follows:

BMI (kg/m2)	Assessment
<18.5	Underweight
18.5 – 29.9	Ideal/healthy weight
25 – 29.9	Overweight
≥ 30	Obese

Obesity is divided into the following three classes:

Class I: BMI between 30.0 and 34.9 kg/m^2
Class II: BMI between 35.0 and 39.9 kg/m^2
Class III: BMI≥40.0 kg/m^2 (morbid obesity)

Waist circumference takes into account deep underlying abdominal fat. Expansion of the waist circumference measurement, while keeping the BMI constant, is considered a more accurate indicator of mortality.

The cut off measurement for a healthy waist circumference varies according to gender. High-risk waist circumferences for men and women are detailed below.

Adult males: Above 101.6 cm (40 in.)
Adult females: Above 88.9 cm (35 in.)

Indications are that an abdominal circumference of about 43 inches and greater in men is likely accompanied by a 50 percent increase in mortality rates compared to an individual with 8 inches less in the stomach. Similarly for women, a 37.5 inch waistline may mean 80 percent greater mortality compared to an individual with about 10 inches less in the waist.

There is also waist to height ratio. rarely used but probably the best of both worlds in that it may be a better predictor of both body fat percentage and visceral fat mass than either BMI or waist circumference. The rule of thumb for this measurement is: *keep your waist less than half your height.*

WHY ARE YOU OVERFAT?

Weight management and body fat reduction do not come easily for everyone. The impact of genetics may be expressed in different ways including appetite control, feelings of fullness, body metabolism, body fat distribution, and eating as a way of coping with stress. The "fat gene" scientifically referred to as FTO (fat mass and obesity associated) is the gene most loosely associated with obesity.

Traditionally, it was felt that genetic disposition explains less than 1% of the difference in fatness between individuals, accounting for a few hundred extra calories of food intake over a year. Over the years, opinions on this matter have changed. Genetic disposition varies considerably among individuals, and the gene effect is now reported as ranging between 25% and as much as 80%. Given the same number of calories as other members of an ad hoc group, the high-rated cases gain significantly more weight than the others because they are so genetically disposed. Simply put, they are born that way (Greger, 2019).

Good indicators of genetic influence include stubborn-fat retention, as evidenced by difficulty in losing weight, overweight parents, and a sustained overweight appearance over most of a lifespan (as much as 80%). Consequently, a strong genetic disposition for obesity will yield less favourable results for traditional programmes of diet and exercise and may result in difficulties in the achievement of reduced weight.

It does not mean that such individuals are forced to live throughout life with that societally less-appreciated look. It means having a greater sense of awareness and working harder to be where you want to be. The inheritance factor is not a reason for resignation. Your fate is not necessarily sealed at birth.

But what about the influence of the mother's condition or that of a surrogate mother who provides the prevailing conditions within the uterus? Indications are that the nurturing condition of the uterus wins out. Obesity of the surrogate mother who carries the fetus would seem to have greater influence than that of the biological mother who supplied the egg. Research data emphasise the importance of preventing obesity and ensuring effective treatment to prevent or minimize the transmission of obesity to future generations.

It appears that this maternal influence can reach as far back as two generations to that of the grandmother. Indications are that your fat level is even affected by what your mother ate during pregnancy. Research data point to animal protein consumed by mothers during pregnancy, increasing the risk of children growing up overweight and potentially increasing their risk of obesity later in life. The actual food intake or exercise regime adopted by the child made no significant difference in outcome; this particular finding may be questioned! To avoid pediatric obesity, weight loss should not be ignored.

If you are frustrated in a struggle with managing obesity, don't lose hope. Remember that gene power is toppled by the power of your fork or spoon. Keep a sense of humour, do not resign yourself to simply believing that it "runs in the family," and meditate on these statements by Michael Greger (2019): "Genes may load the gun, but diet pulls the trigger".

Increasingly, the literature gives weight to a genetic factor in predicting obesity. A good bit of self advice to the individual struggling with the problem is that some people have to work harder than others. . Genetic inheritance for a predisposition for extra weight gain is not an acceptable excuse for personal resignation to the inevitable, so to speak. Let it be a source of intense motivation to put in the extra effort to unseal your fate.

BODY FAT

Traditionally, fat cells are said to remain in the body *forever* and are the biggest enemy in the effort to reduce obesity. The problem is not the addition of new fat cells but rather the fact that they just get bigger and bigger and bigger. Supposedly, the number of fat cells in the human body, whether lean or obese, is established during the childhood and adolescent years. Thereafter, the changes which take place relate to volume and not number. Fat cells increase in size as they take in fatty acids, and they shrink when fatty acids are released from fat storage.

A compilation of notes based upon research/comments on the subject by selected scientists [Dr. Shirisha Avadhanula, Dr Bruce Buchholz, Dr B Burguera and others] provides some interesting information on continuing dialogue in this line of research. The idea that fat cells never "die" would seem to be now regarded as a myth. Approximately 10 percent of fat cells are renewed annually for adults at all ages and levels of body mass index. Fat cell death or its generation rate does not appear to be altered in early obesity onset. There is an indication that numbers of fat cells can be altered through apoptosis [programmed cell death in adults] in various parts of the body. It is possible to see fat cells disintegrate. They do eventually die.

Research indicates an interesting relationship between "berry polyphenols" and the death of fat cells by apoptosis. They provide protection against endotoxins and inhibit a particular enzyme, fatty acid synthase, which is supposedly responsible for making new fat cells. They also appear to be able to imitate fat cell apoptosis [fat death]. Overall, the emerging suggestion is that dietary changes for fat management can include the use of a high intake of berries[blueberries, raspberries, blackberries] and other sources of polyphenols including a vast array of spices, herbs, teas. . Pineapple is also identified as the richest sources of bromelain, found in the stem and core, with tremendous potential for apoptosis,. This is used to get rid of cells that are damaged beyond repair.

The discussion raises the possibility of a slow removal of fat cells, thereby making it more difficult to regain weight. This is a matter of ongoing research.

Fat cells have a mean lifespan of 10 years with 10% undergoing a yearly renewal, thereby maintaining the tight balance of new fat cell formation and the "death" (apoptosis) of older mature cells. Nevertheless, the pre-vailing point of view is that noticeable weight loss results from changes in size of fat cells, with the total number remaining the same. Prolonged obesity can lead to increased fat cell formation without an accompanying apoptosis but with an increase in cell size; a kind of double negative effect in the battle for weight loss.

Body–fat percentage is calculated as the total mass of fat divided by total body weight multiplied by 100. Body fat is generally referred to as adipose tissue; its main role being an energy reserve for the body. A body fat level of 7% with a weight of 180 pounds means that 12.6 pounds of total body weight is fat. Each pound supposedly stores a few thousand calories.

For women, their essential fat is approximately 8%–10%. The essential fat level for men is about 2%–3%. A limit of about 10% is recommended as the minimal for the average individual. With this in mind, a desirable level of 21%–24% for men and 22%–31% for women is recommended, provided they maintain active lifestyles and good eating patterns.

Physical Location of Fat on the Body

Fat on the bodies of men mostly collects above the waist and over the abdominal muscles. Superficial fat under the skin, which accounts for flabby arms, is the source of what is called "cellulite." The loose, pinchable flab on the torso is called "subcutaneous fat."

In contrast, across the midsection soft cavity which contains the intestines, liver, and kidneys, we find the "visceral fat." This type of fat is considered dangerous stuff. It wraps around the organs mentioned and cannot be removed by liposuction, a process in which fat is sucked up from the adipose fat cells from the areas of the back, flanks, and stomach.

The subcutaneous types are assigned to the middle spare tyre and the visceral type is assigned to the fat wrapped around the inner organs.

- High waist circumference is indicative of android (male-type) obesity.
- Android obesity means a greater proportion of body fat in the upper body, especially in the abdomen; described as the "apple" shape
- Gynoid (female-type) obesity means a greater proportion of body fat in the lower body, especially in the hips and thighs. This is described as the "pear" shape

Women are equipped for reproduction by carrying essential fat in their breasts and hips. In general, they have a higher percentage of body fat than men. Their fat storage is subcutaneous before menopause and is concentrated in the "gluteal-femoral" (buttocks, thighs) region. Women, after menopause, and men have their fat storage concentrated in the visceral (abdominal) depot.

Upper Body (Visceral) Fat

The location of fat on your body may, in some circumstances, be more important than the quantity of fat. Just as fat types differ in food, so it is with human body fat. Visceral fat builds up around prominent internal organs in the middle soft section of the human body. It is often referred to as the "killer fat" or "dangerous stuff." The fat around your liver is not the same as the fat around your quadriceps.

Visceral fat coils around and infiltrates your internal organs and presents itself as the bulging "beer belly" in men. The "fat depots" of upper body fat, including the visceral fat referred to above, store and release energy easily and readily for use by the body. The breakdown of fat into fatty acids keeps the blood stream flooded with a high concentration of fat. This increases the potential for serious health problems, including a preponderance of LDL (bad) cholesterol and triglycerides as well as Alzheimer's disease. Fortunately, proper exercise of the muscles leads to a release of enzymes, which extract the dangerous triglycerides and burn them as fuel. Even if weight loss is limited, it is reported that exercise helps to burn visceral fat and build the more desirable muscle in its place. Unfortunately, this type of fat is susceptible to inflammation, which facilitates insulin resistance leading to either pre-diabetes or type 2 diabetes. We then arrive at what is known as "metabolic syndrome," as discussed later in the text. Another related condition of significance is inflamed body tissues accompanied by a narrowing of blood vessels and a raising of blood pressure.

It should be noted that a large waist is not an automatic indication of excessive visceral fat. Similarly, a thin waist does not always signal that the body is in perfect condition. There is a condition known as "thin outside, fat inside" or "TOFI."

Below the Waist (Lower Body) Fat

Fat below the waist behaves very differently. This fat is stored away, causes very little harm to the body, and is used as a last reserve. This fat produces less inflammatory compounds related to LDL concentration and the prospect of cardiovascular damage is much less. Women tend to register lower-body fat storage than men, such as fat hips.

The Fat Colour Scheme

Generally, it is said that there are two forms of fat or adipose tissue: white fat cells that specialise in the storage of chemical energy and calories, and brown cells that burn fat and glucose into energy to generate heat. The latter is considered "good" fat. The capacity to control switching from one to the other, with an emphasis on the more desirable brown, remains an area of active research with possible significance for obesity management. The spice turmeric enhances weight loss since it contains the compound curcumin, which reportedly enhances weight loss by its ability to transform white fat into brown fat and by its regulation of lipid metabolism, preventing the formation of mature fat cells.

For information only, I have also observed a broader categorization of adipose tissue into brown, beige, white subcutaneous, and white visceral cells. White types remain the challenging types in the obesity struggle.

DOES EXCESS FAT MATTER?

In a general sense, there is no indication that a few excess pounds necessarily pose a health risk; however, there is a point where a wakeup call about your personal health is needed, when the pounds and rolls of fat make you feel uncomfortable. The fact is, being overweight or obese *can* and *will* most likely lead to health problems—both physical and emotional.

It may be fun to joke about your being "pleasantly plump" or "just a bit rounded" or "having a little more material for your partner to deal with" and so forth, but you've got to know when the joke is no longer a joke, and it may be worth your while to acknowledge potential or actual health problems!

If you look around and you conclude that you carry a lot more fat on your body than most people around you, it may be that you ought to give some consideration to serious personal reflection. There are cases where rare and unusual health conditions make it almost impossible or very difficult for the individual to achieve effective weight management. Apart from such situations, the obese person must be cautious about having an attitude that the world must accept you as you are and that there are no serious consequences for remaining overweight.

Fats represent, as we see, an active storage facility in the body for materials such as molecules of excess hormones (such as estrogen), fat-soluble vitamins, pollutants, and toxins. The risk factor associated with being overweight comes into play with the shrinkage of body size. Besides the release of fatty acids, these other stored materials also get released. Female body fat, for example, produces some of its own estrogen and stores it. The presence of extra body fat means additional exposure and an increased risk of breast cancer caused by estrogen malfunction.

Some vitamins are absorbed by body fat (adipose tissue) and are not released, possibly leading to vitamin deficiency. Vitamins A, D, E and K appear to be of particular interest. This particular storage aspect of excess fat may lead to vitamin D deficiency in overweight people. Pollutants can be readily released via urination, but some tend to persist in fat tissue, again underscoring the advantages of getting rid of excess fat.

It has been indicated that loss of a single pound of fat represents a kind of self detoxification in that the body is able to use its own filtration system in order to get rid of environmental pollutants which tend to find safe storage in body fat.

It is important to be aware of the fact that excess fat interferes with the effective functioning of the important hormone leptin, which plays a major role in regulating food intake and is directly related to the management of obesity. Without leptin, you can eat to dangerous, uncontrolled levels. It regulates the body's response to signals from the stomach indicating that it is full. More fat cells mean more leptin in circulation and good signal transfer on the quantity eaten; however, while this mechanism works well in lean persons, there is considerable reduction of efficiency in overweight persons. The role of leptin is discussed in greater detail elsewhere in the text.

SUMMARY

This chapter provides lots of general information on body fat. Readers will be able to choose to focus on or ignore various sections based on limited or extended interest in a particular topic. Hopefully, there is enough for a wide range of appetites.

The remaining chapters allow the reader to explore a wide variety of interesting topics which are relevant to the onset of excess body fat and the many initiatives pursued in preventing or treating the condition. The overall presentation is an effort to help the individual achieve and maintain an improved personal appearance, long-term overall health, and ultimately the acquisition of lifestyle habits associated with good human health.

CHAPTER 2
BREAKFAST: HOW IMPORTANT IS THIS MEAL?

OPINIONS VARY SOMEWHAT on the importance of breakfast . There is a long-standing tradition of referring to breakfast as the most important meal of the day. It has even been tied to successful weight loss. The brief overview in this chapter covers some experimental observations and varying conclusions on the subject. It refers to the first meal of the day after not eating overnight.

Greger (2019) provides comprehensive discussion on a wide range of studies relating to breakfast and weight loss. One line of reasoning makes the case that there is strong evidence that eating breakfast is important for weight maintenance, metabolism, and overall good health, that is, regularly eating a substantial morning meal directly affects how fat cells function in the body by changing the activity of genes involved in fat metabolism and insulin resistance.

There is even a suggestion that having breakfast is the "the best kept waist-trimming secret" in the fight against obesity.

At the time of going to bed, insulin levels are flat without any extreme surge. If we arise in the morning and do not "break the fast"—that is, we skip breakfast—blood sugar levels drop and insulin levels drop; however, later in the day and leading up to lunch, there is a strong likelihood of a hunger craze. The typical behavioural response is an increase in the consumption of carbohydrates and not necessarily of the most desirable type of food which assists the weight control effort. Meal skipping guarantees the firing up of sugar cravings and overeating to make up for earlier missed calories with consequences which almost guarantee a continuing condition of excess weight. Inevitably, we arrive at a surge or spike of insulin leading to a "crash" with negative consequences for weight management. Over time, the constant flux (rise and fall) of insulin levels can lead to type 2 diabetes. In essence, habitually skipping breakfast does not appear to be a good idea for individuals aiming to keep off extra weight.

Studies out of prestigious U.S. research institutions, such as Harvard University and the University of Minnesota, give positive indications of clear advantages of eating breakfast. In one study of eating habits and health outcomes of 46,289 women over 6 years, it was found that skipping breakfast was associated with a 20% higher risk of type 2 diabetes compared to individuals who made breakfast a daily habit. The Rhode Island National Weight Control Registry tracked individuals with successful weight loss of at least 30 lb and revealed that one bit of the Holy Grail in the process is that they never skipped breakfast.

There is some evidence that skipping breakfast may be more habitual among women, being even more noticeable among overweight women. Some individuals speak of having difficulty eating first thing in the morning. Working women need take note that occasionally missing breakfast showed an even higher risk level of 54%.

Research referenced in the UK and elsewhere also supports not skipping breakfast as being associated with better glucose control in fat cells of the body. The results from experimentation are not always that clear. Some results show no significant differential effect whatsoever.

When recommended, the emphasis is on the practice of a daily breakfast schedule and eating within an hour or two of waking up. Mere cups of coffee or tea are not a substitute for a meaningful breakfast.

There is a hint that some of the breakfast success stories reported may be funded by cereal manufacturers (that is, bias in design and interpretation of results).

A good breakfast, including a combination of high-quality protein and fats, means a stomach occupied with digestion and avoidance of hunger pangs later in the morning. The inclusion of good vegetable fibre is a plus in many ways. Suggestions will vary with geographical location. In North America, inclusions may be asparagus, broccoli, mushrooms, and a variety of peppers. High-protein options include eggs, peanut butter, low fat cheese, and Greek yogurt. Some nutritionists warn, however, against Greek yogurt. Reportedly, Greek yogurt can cause some less-than-ideal side effects, including inflammatory issues with some individuals.

There is caution with respect to fruit for breakfast as is a common habit for some persons. This should be limited to one piece of fruit to avoid blood sugar spikes. Whole fruit is associated with lots of fibre but usually contains substantial amounts of fructose (fruit sugar). In this regard, possible safe fruit choices include apples with lots of fibre in the skin and with a low glycemic index, as well as grapefruit and berries. If your personal battle of the bulge is a big one, leave out the fruit.

On the matter of blood sugar control, a major recommendation on dietary control for any meal is the avoidance of bread, in particular, white bread. The reasoning behind this is discussed at length under the heading of "wheat belly" in Chapter 5. Indications are that there may well be a measurable decline in bread consumption in recent times; however, the problem lies in greatly improved efficiency in refined milling of wheat, resulting in a mining of nutrients, especially wheat germ oil which is subsequently sold back to the general population by the vitamin industry as vitamin E.

TIMING IS SIGNIFICANT

Typically, in many societies, breakfast is the smallest meal of the day; we seem to be hungrier in the evening after our cumulative daily activity. The matter of our circadian rhythm apparently comes into play. The hunger naturally peaks at about 8:00 p.m. with its lowest level at about 8:00 a.m., even after many hours overnight without food.

Colbert (2016) references an interesting study from Tel Aviv University involving 93 obese women assigned to eat the same foods (totalling 1040 calories) over a 12-week period but with differences in time of consumption. One half of the participants were assigned a small breakfast (200 calories), a medium lunch (300 calories), and a big (700 calories) dinner. The other half consumed their calories in the reverse order. Reportedly, the results were "staggering"; the big-breakfast group lost an average of 17.8 pounds and 3 inches off the waistline over 12 weeks, compared to 7.3 pounds and 1.4 inches off the waistline for the other group (Greger, 2019).

The difference was timing.

It was found that the big-breakfast group had significantly lower levels of ghrelin, an appetite depressant, which generally leads to greater food satisfaction and a reduced desire for intermittent snacking during the day. On this matter of timing, Colbert (2016) writes:

> The study conclusively showed just how important timing is to weight loss. Within three months, the "big breakfast" group proved that fact by losing almost three times as much weight as the "big dinner" group in spite of the fact that they had the same number of calorie intakes each day.

Similarly, in comparison to the one meal a day groups (morning or evening), the morning intake group fared better at weight loss.

The prevailing conclusion favours a hearty morning meal followed by a lighter lunch and dinner. The idea is that this pattern burns twice as many calories compared to heavier meals later in the day, regardless of the fact that the same total number of calories are consumed in the two different intake patterns. One explanation is that metabolism is in high gear in the morning, implying the body has a greater capacity to burn fat for energy.

According to registered dietician and medical writer Lindsey DeSoto (2017), "Breakfast earned its title as the most important meal of the day back in the 1960s after American nutritionist, Adelle Davis, suggested that to keep fit and avoid obesity, one should 'eat breakfast like a king, lunch like a prince, and dinner like a pauper.'" The royal titles refer to portion size (calories per meal), with King being the heaviest meal.

Research focussed on the "king–prince–pauper" versus "pauper–prince–king" comparative consumption pattern is interesting. In each group, the total consumption for all three meals was the same. The result followed the predominant pattern indicated so far: the morning-slanted group lost more than twice as much weight, in addition to slimming about an extra two inches off their waistline. By the end of the 12-week study, the king-prince-pauper group lost 11 more pounds (19 pounds lost compared to 8 despite eating the same number of calories). That's the power of chronobiology, the power of our circadian rhythms. (Greger, 2019)

Regardless of the percentage distribution of calories by meal pattern, the bigger-breakfast group takes the prize for dramatically increased weight loss. The lesson from all this is: eat more in the morning than in the evening if the goal is to lose weight.

The consistency in these findings helps us to understand another popular variant of the phrase above: "Eat breakfast yourself, share lunch with a friend, and give dinner away to your enemy." In short, skip dinner rather than breakfast.

Interesting commentaries suggest that most of the claimed benefits of eating breakfast are derived from observational studies without any proof of cause cum effect. Indications are that there may be reduced risk for heart disease, abdominal obesity diabetes, and other related health conditions. Data relating to some 30,000 North Americans show that skipping breakfast may result in deficiencies relating to foliate, calcium, iron, and vitamins A, B, C, D; possibly also a disruption of circadian rhythms. In essence, the summary position is one of complexity (DeSoto, 2022).

On the matter of meal-consumption timing, late-night or evening snacks are also concerns. Indications are that evaluation must take place within an overall calorie-intake plan for the entire day. If night snacking is a habit, control mid-morning and other snacks to accommodate the habit. The after-dark snacks must also be healthy; apple slices and peanut butter do receive favourable mention.

Cumulative research also suggests that we pay attention to the idea of "dinner at 6." Indications are that eating dinner at 6 p.m. can ultimately lead to burning twice as much fat compared to eating large amounts of calories later in the day. This facilitates better synchronisation of the body clock accompanied by suppression of the hunger hormone, ghrelin, and increasing the effect of the satiety hormone, leptin.

SUMMARY

Some caution is suggested at reaching hard and fast conclusions about the breakfast issue. The fact is that many writers on nutrition in weight loss management strongly recommend that breakfast is an important meal for effective control of calorie intake and maximising metabolic activity. A not-so-favourable point of view is a suggestion that a number of positive responses on breakfast are coming out of research which is very much influenced by the fact that research funding originated from cereal makers. There is also a body of research, some of it at the university level, which regards the morning breakfast theory as a myth. It is reported that similar studies from several universities have indicated no significant differences in weight loss between groups which ate or skipped breakfast (Dr. Oz, 2020; Harvard Medical School, 2020).

Whether this is a myth or scientific reality is simply not clear. There is no evidence to suggest that having breakfast has negative results.

CHAPTER 3
WATER: DISCOVER THE MIRACLE OF NATURE

MY PERSONAL STRUGGLE with weight management and my willingness to try various recommendations led me to the discovery of the miraculous ways in which just water can contribute to weight management in the human body.

The suggestion to drink lots of water is quite common. I am convinced, however, that most people do not understand the power of water in the pursuit of good health. I say this because my efforts at persuading adults to follow what I understand to be an ancient Chinese practice, as circulated on WhatsApp for example, of water down the hatch first thing in the morning has been met with great surprise by individuals deciding to give it a try. Indeed, when I first caught on, I was surprised. Then, later on, I learnt to apply strategic water intake at various times, such as after a late-night dinner, to achieve the ultimate objective of improved transit through the large intestine.

Numerous references in the literature from weight loss experts advise drinking more water to fast-track weight loss. I have attempted to cover the matter with some degree of thoroughness, emphasis being placed on the individual management of water intake.

BASIC METABOLIC RATE: WHAT DOES WATER DO?

Put simply, metabolism describes all the chemical reactions in the body which keeps it alive and functioning. The rate of metabolism is the amount of energy used per unit of time. Basic metabolic rate (BMR) is the amount of energy (the number of calories) used or burnt daily as the body performs basic life-sustaining functions, such as breathing. A calorie is a unit of energy in nutrition. Calories refer to the energy people get from food and drink consumed and the energy they use in physical activity. It is a measure of energy expenditure and of stored energy. For example, exercise causes an increase in BMR. The higher the BMR, the more calories are burned.

Research indicates that drinking water has a tremendous effect on the body's metabolic rate. A 30% increase in metabolic rate has been demonstrated for both men and women who drink two cups of water (Vij & Joshi, 2013). Similarly, the importance of avoiding dehydration is demonstrated by the fact that even 1% dehydration can cause a significant drop in metabolism.

Water is involved in every possible type of cellular process in the body and there is a wide range of chemical processes affected. Cell dehydration decreases the level of activity related to glucose uptake as induced by insulin, an important process highlighted throughout this book as it affects the spike in blood sugar levels. In contrast, adequate hydration enhances efficiency and also affects general body metabolism.

WATER CONTENT AND TIMING OF FOOD INTAKE

In a more general sense, water is considered important to general gut health, flushing out toxins, and helping to eliminate excess fat from the body. Water is absorbed by the intestines and circulates as fluids, delivering oxygen and nutrients to cells. It takes away waste materials which are eliminated in urine. There must be a sufficiency of water passing through the system for effective flushing. There is a popular saying among water enthusiasts: the emphasis being to drink, drink more, and more!

Chinese proverbs on the matter of drinking warm or cold water seem to suggest that warm water facilitates contraction of the intestines with expedition to waste elimination. Warm water is said to activate the digestive tract, and there is the general acceptance that water does work as a lubricant along the length of the digestive tract, providing both hydration and the flushing out of toxins for better health.

Timing water intake has its advantages. Drinking water before a meal brings on a feeling of satiety and reduces appetite and calorie intake; however, it would seem to be most applicable in middle-aged and older adults. There are indications of increased weight loss by as much as 2 kg (4.4 lb) over a 12-week period. As much as 44% more weight loss has been achieved with a group of overweight and obese participants who drank water before each meal compared to another group that did not consume water. The water consumers reduced calorie intake by about 9% (200 calories) on average on a daily basis.

There is, however, some variation of thought on this matter. There also exists a point of view that drinking water with meals does not necessarily cut down on food intake. A point is being made that there is some difference with water in food, such as soup or a blended meal, as compared to water alongside the meal, the latter appearing to be much more effective in achieving a feeling of fullness and leading to reduced intake as a result of reduced stomach space. However, it would appear that water consumed within (not separated) from the actual food "is more closely related to a slimmer waist." (Greger, 2019) Supposedly, people misunderstand thirst for hunger and reach for snacks to consume. Grabbing a glass of no-calorie water instead of traditional snack food can help to reduce the intake of unwanted calories. Always remember: water is 100% calorie free. This is especially important for individuals attempting to give up sodas and juices in exchange for water at mealtimes.

Research involving obese men and women who drank 2 cups of water three times a day, a half hour before meals (that is, over and above their regular water intake) lost an average of 5 pounds more body fat in 12 weeks compared to a control group. In general, the half-hour period before meal consumption seems to be the dominant recommendation.

A long term, comprehensive Harvard study involving the review of diets and health of over 100,000 medical personnel for decades demonstrated over the long-term that increasing water intake per se was independently and significantly associated with less weight gain.

Similar results have been observed among school children. The provision of water fountains and appropriate classroom instruction suggests a 31% reduction in obesity. The water advantage is evident with weight management with obese and overweight children, a matter of interest to parents and guardians.

Reduced calorie intake can range between 13%–20% (more than 100 calories) or as much as 44% for overweight men with participants who took 2 cups of water before each meal. There is a space replacement effect within the digestive tract giving a sense of fullness. In addition, it does appear that water also accounts for a metabolic or fat-burning effect. Sparkling, high-fizz beverages seem to also have the same and perhaps an even better effect.

Drinking water before breakfast is a growing trend. As much as 13% reduction in calories has been recorded as a result of drinking water before breakfast. A common recommendation in the literature is to begin each day with 8 oz of hot water mixed with the juice of half a lemon, together with two servings of fibre-rich vegetables. There is a recommendation that apple cider vinegar (ACV) can be substituted for lemon juice.

While there are many advisories on warm water, especially in the morning, there is also the suggestion that cold (refrigerator-temperature) water is much more effective in boosting metabolic rate and burning calories.

Ways of raising the metabolic rate are critical in achieving weight loss. It is directly affected by level of hydration. The article "The Link Between Dehydration and Metabolism" in *Wellness Magazine* states that over 70% of muscle consists of water and there is a deficiency in capacity for energy generation in a dehydrated state.

My personal experience with water first thing in the morning is very positive. I have also found that the occasional use of water without adding either lemon juice or ACV still had a positive result. My cumulative experience with drinking water in relation to weight control enables me to advise to drink water simply because it is good and effective. I would add keep water and a glass visible in a frequently traversed location and drink without wanting to drink. From personal experience, here are four occasions to drink water:

1. First thing in the morning, drink one to two glasses of water.
2. Drink one to glasses about 15–20 minutes before eating anything solid.
3. You get the feeling for a bowel movement (BM).; Experience lends some confidence that a glass of water makes it less likely to be a difficult one!
4. Dined out and had a heavy meal, or feeling stuffed and uncomfortable. To avoid these feelings, drink the first glass of cold or warm water; a second glass at about 15–20 minutes at the restaurant or on arriving at your next stop; a third glass in about another 20–30 minutes. If no BM action, a fourth glass ought to bring the much-needed relief; a marvellous experience of relief especially before turning in to bed at nights.

A major lesson being touted here is the tremendous positive effect of drinking water consistently throughout the day.

It is of interest to note the rapidity with which water works on the system; it commences within 10 minutes and reaches a maximum burn of 24 calories within 90 minutes. Take note that a tall glass of plain, cheap, and safe tap water four times during the day has the potential to burn an extra 100 calories.

Purposeful, routine consumption of water makes it significant on both sides of the calorie balance equation; both *in* and *out*. Filling space on the *in* side, such as drinking water just before a meal, means a reduced calorie intake.

In general, water consumption before eating does appear to reduce calorie intake; this may slow a bit with age. From personal experience, I am inclined to recommend strongly that the latter possibility be ignored. Positive effects are definitely projected.

It's important to remember that in the pursuit of effective weight management that every bit helps. In one case, a study indicated that water before meals led to average of 75 fewer calories at each meal. If we calculate this advantage at least once every day, 75 x 365 means at least 27000 calories on the *in* side in a single year; definitely worthy of serious consideration. Many individuals have the problem of late-night raids on the refrigerator because of a feeling of hunger. Research has shown that a single glass of water can eliminate the feeling of night hunger pangs in many instances.

SUGARY DRINKS AND DIET SODAS

Greger (2019) makes an impacting statement:

> The primary reason that the Centers for Disease Control and Prevention, U.S. Department of Agriculture, American Medical Association, American Diabetes Association, American Heart Association and American Academy of Pediatrics all recommend drinking water for weight management is as a replacement for sugary beverages. Swapping just one sweetened beverage or beer a day with water is associated with a lower incidence of obesity over time.

Long term weight gain in some populations averages about 3.2 lb (1.45 kg) every 4 years. It is suggested that increased daily intake of 1 cup of water can reduce this amount by 0.23 lb; this figure increases more than 400% to 1.1 lb when water is substituted for sugar-sweetened drinks. Additional substitutes are low-fat milk and tea. Daily substitution of sugary drinks by an individual can account for a reduction of some 235 calories a day on average.

Beware of diet sodas. Studies in which water replaced diet sodas gave plain water the edge. As with herbal tea, the concentration of dissolved substances is about 12 times that of plain tap water. Plain water on an empty stomach would seem to be the best path to follow. It is of interest to note that results of a Harvard study demonstrated that the risk of obesity increased by 31 percent as a result of drinking one soft drink a day, diet or regular. [Swap & Drop Diet, New Canadian No-Diet Revolution. 2012]

A good bit of advice is not to buy and, therefore, keep out of sight what you wish to avoid drinking (or eating); remove the temptation.

QUANTITY OF WATER INTAKE

The composition of water in the human body ranges between 50% and 75%. Recommendations on water consumption appear to have been somewhat random over a long period; the classic being eight eight-ounce glasses per day for almost everyone, or about 2 litres (1 litre equals 0.0296 fl oz) for men and 1.6 litres for women. Quantities are to be increased if caffeine (tea, coffee, chocolate) is taken.

Changes are indicated in recent years with some relevance to individual cases. Size, body weight, and activity levels are increasingly taken into consideration; for example, between half an ounce and one ounce of water for each pound of body weight each day. One male versus female recommendation is as follows.

Assuming moderate physical activity at moderate ambient temperatures, an example of recommended daily water intake for females is 7 cups (ages 9–13), 8 cups (14–18), and 9 cups (19+). The corresponding figures for males are 8, 11, and 13 cups. This means about one cup every waking hour for adults. The advisory limit appears to be no more than 3 cups in an hour, the projected limit which can be efficiently handled by the kidneys.

An additional aspect determines the quantity of water needed for weight management. Heavier people actually need to consume more water; for example, a man of average height weighing 210 lb may have a requirement of 4 cups more water than an individual weighing 160 lb.

Absolutely "yes" is the indicated response to the potential for drinking too much water. Beyond AA3 cups of water per hour, there is a risk of depleting the water supply in the human brain and with lethal consequences (Greger, 2019).

If you need assistance in developing a habit of drinking water sufficiently, there is an App for that; it reminds the individual to drink at preselected intervals.

At least one group of researchers suggests caution. In general, extra water hydration is expected to curtail hunger, flush fat promoting toxins, and fire up cellular metabolism, all of which contribute positively to weight management. However, somewhat recently, researchers appear to have uncovered new scientific findings which suggest that there may be a negative side to large intakes of water in the case of women who facing issues relating to bloat, fatigue and indigestion The result may be a worsening of symptons and recognisable weight gain..

They noted that 80% of women over 40 have a deficiency of stomach acid, a situation aggravated by lifestyle circumstances such as stress, excessive alcohol consumption and use of varying medications, all of which impair the acid producing function of the stomach. In such circumstances, further dilution of the already limited acid supply, especially drinking water before and during a meal, can result in weakening the digestive capacity of the stomach. This means potential malnutrition since an ample supply of stomach acid is essential for breaking down and absorption of protein and almost one third of essential vitamins and minerals.

Stomach acid is also significant in the body release of bile. Insufficient stomach acid means inadequate bile release and lowered capacity of the body to digest fat which then ends up being stored instead of being burnt to provide fuel for energy supply.

The complication is even more far-reaching. Low stomach acid can lead to digestive malfunctioning which negatively affects nutrient absorption and the general performance of critical weight management organs. We learn in later chapters the importance of insulin and the pancreas in the balancing of metabolic activity.

The same scenario plays out; the pancreas and the liver, our "slimming organs," jump into the fray, pumping out digestive enzymes to balance the supply situation. This has a temporary or stop-gap effect. These organs tend to function to meet the requirements for individual meals or snacks. Frequent malfunctioning of the metabolic amphitheatre in the stomach diminishes their primary performance capacity with respect to burning fat, flushing toxins, and regulating blood sugar. Reportedly, stomach acid levels correctly managed can result in a melting of 7 pounds and loss of several inches a week.

A NOTE ON WATER FASTING AND WATER-BASED DIETS

Water fasting is a kind of fasting during which only water is consumed. It is tried for various reasons including religion, health benefits, before a medical procedure, detoxing, and to lose weight.

Approximately 2 3 liters are consumed daily over a 24 to 72 hour period and can lead to a loss of up to 2 pounds (0.9 kg) per day. Longer periods are not recommended without medical supervision. The preparatory phase may take as long as 4 days. The post-fast phase, like for all fasts, must be managed regarding food and liquid intake. This is important to avoid refeeding syndrome, a potentially fatal condition in which the body undergoes rapid variation in fluid and electrolyte levels. An associated negative result is orthostatic hypotension, a drop in blood pressure leading to the individual becoming dizzy or lightheaded and with a risk of fainting. The process is not recommended for persons with gout, diabetes, or eating disorders.

Research has shown that water fasting can improve the body's sensitivity to insulin and leptin thereby making it more effective in health management. Improved insulin sensitivity means greater efficiency in regulating blood sugar levels. Leptin sensitivity relates to the body being better able to process hunger signals, thereby reducing the risk of obesity.

Lemon Water Detox

One commentary expresses the view that lemon water cannot detox or cleanse the body as is sometimes touted and that it is merely a fad or quick fix diet; it has no fibre which is necessary for the cleansing process. The added benefits of lemon do not include any detoxification prowess but can add small quantities of vitamin C, antioxidants, and potassium. A kind of accessory recommendation to the early morning intake discussed above is one of lemon juice and filtered water; the gut benefit indicated is increased stomach acidity for killing undesirable pathogens before they leave the stomach (Vysohlid, 2019). One point of view, however, is that lemon acids "thin out sludgy bile"—all for the sake of improved elimination. There is also the simple commentary that the pectin present in lemon simply helps to suppress food cravings and assist in keeping off the unwanted pounds.

Cucumber Water and Mint Water

Benefits indicated from cucumber and mint in water bottles on desks in offices and so forth include the facts that cucumbers are rich in potassium; the electrolyte reduces salt in the bloodstream enabling good blood pressure. Mint-flavoured water is a source of vitamin A and antioxidants.

Apple Cider Vinegar: Early-Morning Addition
to Water, Detox, and Weight Control

Vinegar is referred to as a centuries' old treatment for obesity and an established remedy for diabetes. In some respects, there would seem to be a scarcity of formal research distinct from anecdotal commentaries, many of which can be quite compelling on the detox capability of ACV. There has been some work on its relevance in the treatment of diabetes. Research has shown a positive effect of ACV in the treatment of persons with hyperlipidemia, that is, high blood–fat levels.

There are numerous references to the use of ACV in weight control and other health-promoting initiatives. ACV differs from other kinds of vinegar because of the way it is processed: slow fermentation, low heat, and minimal processing, thereby preserving the minerals and enzymes from the apples. Reportedly, it has been used for detoxification, dietary purposes, and a host of other reasons. It carries a reputation as a kind of healing elixir over thousands of years. In the context of detoxification, the raw, unfiltered ACV which contains "the mother" (seen as murky or cloudy settlement) is said to contain good gut bacteria, vitamins, minerals, and enzymes. The settlement material contains pectin, a prebiotic fibre which feeds and increases activity of our good or beneficial gut bacteria.

A few research reports reference the use of ACV in water as the first intake substance on mornings in relation to weight management. I have used this mixture over fairly long periods, intermittently, with cold or warm water. The treatment does facilitate larger-than-normal bowel releases; in some cases, at least three times for the day. This result is an obvious positive contribution to improved health. I must add, however, that I have experienced almost the same result at times with just plain tap water. It does appear that the quantity of water imbibed is significant. One learns to drink it regardless of the feeling to do so. I have recommended this early morning water intake to other persons, most of whom are impressed by its elimination facilitation and with absolutely no regrets.

I recall one case in which I had to tell my friend who was being introduced to the benefits of drinking water for health purposes to keep drinking; this was her first trial and the request to just keep drinking went on from breakfast time in the morning to well into the night with no results (no elimination). Late in the night, I kept urging my fried to keep the faith. I sent her a message: "To keep [the Rock of] Gibraltar moving, I suggest you get down first thing in the morning the equivalent of two whisky glasses to kickstart the day… you got a lining to lubricate."

The next morning, by about 9 a.m., I got a response in coded language: "I have just come back from the delivery room… I have delivered about 7 lb 8 oz… a baby boy. I am sure you'd be happy to hear safe delivery. Thank you very much, Dad."

Perhaps a bit of exaggeration on the weight; neither was the paternal ascription very welcome. However, I was happy to have made one more convert to adequate water intake early in the morning, in the struggle to achieve improved gut health. Early-morning water intake is also recommended with lemon juice; one reason provided is that the acidity kills pathogens before they leave the stomach, helping to keep the body healthy.

My use of the word "miracle" at the beginning of the section is not by accident. On the strategic use of water, there are lessons to be learnt in the occasional timing of use to maintain gut management. Regardless of the time of day but especially after a meal late in the evening or whenever you get that feeling of "I want to go" but cannot get easy traction, two whisky glasses of pure water can work wonders in about 20–25 minutes. The lining of the small intestine absorbs the flow, and elimination seldom fails the drinker.

Some interesting research has been referenced from Japan. Significant weight losses were recorded with persons on both high (2 tablespoons per day) and low (1 tablespoon per day) daily doses of ACV. Weight losses reported approximated 1 pound per month for the low dosage and 5 pounds for the high-dosage group. The low cost of achieving such progress (pennies per day) was noted. There was a definite reduction of visceral (the killer) fat that builds up around internal organs and is evident with bulging bellies, and also subcutaneous fat (cellulite), which accounts for flabby arms.

ACV appears to have had a definite effect on AMP-activated protein kinase (AMPK activation), a type of enzyme involved in body mechanisms switching from fat storage to fat burning. Build-up of the fat-burning activity switch was almost three times more with persons taking the ACV treatment compared to placebo participants.

In reading this book you would have achieved the important awareness of blood sugar spikes in fat storage and weight control. Spikes are temporarily high blood glucose levels that occur soon after eating. It is normal for glucose level to rise a small amount after eating, with or without diabetes; however, if the rise is too high, this can contribute to serious health problems. Research data has shown a 23% reduction in spiking when 2 teaspoons of vinegar (not necessarily ACV) accompany a high-glycemic meal. This meant improved blood sugar and insulin responses. The interesting results benefitted from research work in Greece which showed that the consumption of vinegar improves the uptake of blood sugar by our muscles.

Also noted was an accompanying feeling of satiety or fullness. These facts partly explain the advantages of cultural cuisine involving the addition of vinegar with white rice, white bread, and potato salad.

The general safe recommendation for taking ACV appears to be 2 tablespoons a day, preferably split into two or even three doses; that is, 2 teaspoons per meal and with food. Other possibilities include addition to side salads or even adding it to tea with some lemon juice.

ACV is now advertised as included in "gummies" and other popular formulations including sugar-free, sour free, and vegan (Nordic formulation).

CRYSTAL/STRUCTURED WATER AND WEIGHT MANAGEMENT

Various claims of benefits for human health with the use of structured or "hexagonal" water have been put forward.. One theory is that the molecules have a higher electrical charge which enhances cell functioning. Oxygen absorption is improved with the advantage of a more efficient immune system. Improved intracellular hydration optimizes mineral and nutrient absorbtion. at the cellular level. On the market is a range of bottles with "natural" crystals which manufacturers advertise as carrying unique healing power. Claims are that drinking 2–3 litres per day results in bodily transformation and a range of health benefits, including weight loss in excess of 20 pounds over 6 month period. Bottled and tap water are referred to as "dead" or "lifeless."

In a more general sense, the use of structured water is said to include improved digestion, elimination of constipation and an improvement of gut microbiology, all of which help to promote weight loss. [https://mayu-water.com]

No reported plausible scientific explanations exist to support the concept of structured water. Timothy Schmidt (2022), the research director of the School of Chemistry at the University of New South Wales, says these claims are made by "snake-oil merchants" who "use scientific-sounding words that are generally meaningless and are at best based on misinterpretations and abuses…"

SUMMARY

Adequate hydration is regarded as one of the keys to effective weight loss. What is quite clear is that it is an area of weight management that can be easily overlooked. The content of this chapter emphasizes the point that it is a fatal error to underestimate the miraculous importance of water hydration in the pursuit of successful weight management. Unlike many weight-loss interventions, water is cost-free.

Remember: *start your day with one, preferably two, glasses of water—*cold, warm, and with or without various suggested additions. You are guaranteed to see the magic! However, do not entertain the idea that this habit, in and by itself, will correct the problem of individual obesity.

CHAPTER 4
DIGESTION: THE SEARCH FOR ENERGY—CARBOHYDRATES, STARCHES, SUGARS, AND PROTEINS

I MUST STATE at the outset that I found the content of this and the next chapter to be the most difficult body of knowledge to pull together for a broad-based audience. But! it had to be done, and apart from the very fascinating Chapter 7 on the microbiome, the material in these two chapters may well be the most important for the reader who is concerned with managing obesity. The content covers the basics of the food we consume, what happens when we eat (digestion), and what ought to happen but what can go wrong and with a host of consequences.

This chapter also provides an early introduction to a single most important word, *insulin*, which lies at the heart of chemical and biological processes taking place along the grand canal, leading from the entry at the mouth to the anal exit. It is a kind of orchestral conductor or grandmaster which largely determines the weight outcome—that is, the potential problem of excessive or abnormal body fat and numerous related health issues.

In a wholesome sense, the digestive processes which take place along the grand canal are by no means simple; they include ingestion, propulsion, mechanical digestion, chemical digestion, absorption, and defaecation.

BASIC DIGESTION: CARBOHYDRATES IN HUMAN NUTRITION

A simple approach to understanding digestion is to regard it, in large part, as the process by which the body breaks down what goes into the mouth as food and utilizes two core activities: physical or mechanical (pulverisation) action, together with chemical treatment. It is all done within what is known as the alimentary canal. The small and large intestines in human beings measure a total of about 25 feet. This lengthy passageway provides time and space for food breakdown and the absorption of water and nutrients; the end products are absorbable and can be used by the body. The passageway also relates to the elimination of food residue. It is to be noted that deficiencies in either of these two processes have a direct effect on the obesity problem which *is* the focus of this book.

CARBOHYDRATES: A MAJOR NUTRIENT GROUP

It is important to understand the nature of the various food types as we deal with the sustenance of human life and maintaining day-to-day good health. *Issues of excess fat deposits and obesity are rooted, in the first instance, in what we put into our mouths as food.*

There are three major nutrient groups in the human diet: carbohydrates, fats, and proteins. All three are relevant in coming to grips with the obesity problem; however, you will become aware that two of them, carbohydrates and fats, hold centre stage in the consciousness of the individual struggling with excess weight management.

The story of excessive body fat commences with the consumption of both carbohydrates and fats, especially the former. We focus our discussion on carbohydrates for a start; members of this group are categorised as "complex" or "simple," as illustrated in the listing of the associated sugars hereunder.

There are also three types of carbohydrates, and they vary in chemical structure: monosaccharides, disaccharides, and trisaccharides. A simplified listing is as follows:

Monosaccharides	Disaccharides
Based on 1 unit of sugar	Based on 2 units of sugar
i.e., simple Sugars	glucose, fructose, galactose,
e.g. lactose, glucose	sucrose = glucose+ fructose; commonly used sugars;

Trisaccharides include a carbohydrate with three monosaccharides linked together; for example, raffinose, which is found in plants and is composed of glucose, fructose, and galactose.

There is also the more complex category of Polysaccharides

Complex carbohydrates, *many* units of sugar joined together; aka polymers i.e., repeating units or chains of monomers); e.g. starch, glycogen, triglycerides

Take note that these different sugars get different treatments in the digestive process along the alimentary canal.

In digestion, the simple monosaccharides readily pass through the wall of the small intestine. The other two types must be broken down into simpler sugars by the appropriate digestive enzymes. For example:

- Starch (rice and potatoes) is broken down into disaccharides by amylase found in saliva
- Lactose (milk) is broken down by lactase
- Sucrose (cane sugar) is broken down by sucrase
- Maltose (in grains) is broken down by maltose
- All the enzyme action takes us towards the simpler monosaccharide products which can then pass through the small intestine.

Wherever the digestive process commences in the structural chain of carbohydrates, the fundamental concept to remember is that the body's objective is to get it all down to sugar. I remember this as: "SOB; IT IS SUGAR."

I also urge you to take special note of one of the three carbohydrate groups: starches. The members of this group are made up of complex, long chains of glucose, an important sugar, and are referred to as polysaccharides.

Keep in mind four important words: carbohydrates, starches, sugar, and glucose. Understanding the implications of the quantity consumed and in what form will help an individual to consciously face up to and manage the problem of obesity and a host of other health-related issues along the way.

Our understanding of the obesity problem means that we need to take a look at the two-way classification of carbohydrates: simple and complex.

Complex Carbohydrates

Complex carbohydrates are composed of long, complex chains of molecules and are sourced from foods such as nuts, vegetables, whole grains, peas, beans, and brown rice, and also from starchy food staples known as "ground provision" in some countries: yams, dasheen, cassava, potatoes, and so forth. Other familiar, highly consumed sources are bread, rice, pasta, corn, wheat, and potatoes. They are harder for the body to break down with a resulting more gradual increase in blood sugar compared to simple carbohydrates.

Simple Carbohydrates

Simple carbs include raw sugar, brown sugar, corn syrup, high-fructose corn syrup (HFCS), glucose, fructose, and sucrose. In the management of obesity on a personal level, it is very important to take note of the following sources: candy, ice cream, white bread, pizza, and sodas. This is the group from which you are most likely to feel a sudden sugar rush in the body when consumed.

Despite all the structural complexity, when broken down (I repeat: *when*), both simple and complex carbohydrates get to what is called glucose, the major source of fuel or energy for body functions.

Simple carbohydrates break down into glucose at a rate faster rather than complex carbohydrates. They are a bigger factor in driving weight gain compared to calories and protein, which actually help to slow both digestion and the balancing of blood sugar! Refining strips carbs of their nutrient-dense casings and leaves a simple carbohydrate chain which the body sees as glucose.

The calorie-based management procedure for controlling obesity is discussed in a later chapter.

STARCHES

Facing the obesity problem requires a super consciousness of problems related to starch consumption.

In general, starch represents a structural assembly or bonding of a single type of molecule and is produced by most plants via the well-known process of photosynthesis in plants. Glucose is a combination of carbon, hydrogen, and oxygen, and we get the structure called carbohydrate. Starch is glucose stored; for example, in grains of wheat, cereals, bread, pasta, rice, corn sweet potatoes, grains, and starchy vegetables. The human body digests starch in the process of getting at glucose as a source of energy. Cells in the body derive their energy from chemical reactions of glucose, a process referred to as aerobic respiration.

It is important to understand what happens when we consume and digest starchy foods. *Remember*: starch is the other member of, together with sugar, my declared SOB cousins. Both are converted to glucose, a sugar. Starchy products (rice, roti, bread, and potatoes) are core dietary items of the majority of the population in most lesser-developed countries and among lower socioeconomic groups. On a day-to-day basis, lots of sugar in popular foods is consumed.

Resistant Starches

All starches are not equal. There is a group classified as "resistant starches"; their molecules resist digestion, functioning somewhat like fibre, and tend to provide increased feelings of fullness (satiation) when consumed. The result is a reduction of caloric intake, thereby facilitating weight loss.

They do not get digested easily and travel far within the digestive tract, almost unchanged, through the small intestine and into the large intestine where fermentation may take place and where they turn into short chain fatty acids which can be absorbed or used by intestinal bacteria.

Here, they act as a prebiotic and contribute to the formation of good gut bacteria which improves glycemic control. Glycemic refers to the effect that food has on blood sugar levels after consumption; discussed later on in the chapter. Benefits include that fullness feeling referred to above, a decrease in cholesterol, prevention of constipation, and a reduced risk of colon cancer. It is said that this group of starches "fill you up without filling you out!"

Sources of resistant starches include potatoes (cooked and cooled); rice; green bananas (when ripe, the starch changes to regular starch); plantains; cashews; whole grains, including oats and barley; and various legumes, such as beans, peas, and lentils. Note that the cooking and cooling process facilitates conversion to the resistant type of carbohydrates, such as with potatoes and rice. White beans and lentils are reportedly the highest in resistant starch.

THE SUGAR STORY

As you read on it will become increasingly obvious why I keep referring to sugar as the "SOB" of fighting the battle of excess body fat and obesity. You will never stop hearing that it is necessary to reduce or carefully manage the intake of sugar. I have no doubt that by the time you get to the end of this book, if not before, you may wish to add a few more colourful, descriptive words for impact effect!

This is the time to get you, the reader, to place firmly in your consciousness *three* words: carbohydrates, starch, and sugar. Get to know and understand them; let them, especially carbohydrates and sugar, forever be a major focus of your consciousness in your battle with obesity. Do this or fail in your struggle!

In this regard, successful weight management demands an understanding of what I choose to call the "sugar story" and an understanding of two "S" words: sugar and starch—my two SOB cousins!

Widely variable levels of carbohydrates are present in almost everything we eat; they all contain a form of sugar going by a variety of names, such as sucrose (table sugar), lactose in milk, and fructose in fruit. Keep in mind that carbohydrates vary in the sugars they carry and the ease or speed with which they give up the sugar when consumed. For purposes of immediate illustration of this important principle, pineapple yields its sweetness faster than grapefruit; a slice of white bread raises your blood sugar faster than a coarse grain (full-of-fibre) cracker. This explains the rush or surge of sugar we sometimes feel when we consume some foods like ice cream.

Insulin: The Glucose-Insulin Interaction

We have already established that via digestion both simple and complex carbohydrates turn into digested glucose (blood sugar) which is the main fuel burnt for energy by our cells. There are alternative destinations with respect to what happens to digestive sugars. They will be used as fuel immediately, stored, or eliminated.

One alternative route, so to speak, is storage in the liver and muscles as glycogen, a multi-unit structure (polysaccharide, combining glucose [a monosaccharide] molecules) and end up being deposited as fat. It has the potential to break down and supply glucose as energy if a supply is not forthcoming in the body at any time.

Effective management of excess fat is aided by an understanding of the significant role played by insulin. It is responsible for stabilization, transportation, and storage in the process of blood sugar management. It regulates blood sugar levels, promotes fat storage, and even helps in the breakdown of fats and proteins.

Another important body organ, the pancreas, comes into the picture with respect to the role of insulin and the management of digestive outcomes. It is a gland in the abdominal cavity where it secretes hormones as part of the body's endocrine system. The endocrine system is a messenger system comprising feedback loops of hormones released by internal glands of an organism into the circulatory system involved in regulating target organs, such as the thyroid gland, pituitary gland, or pancreas. Its significant health function is its role in the conversion of food intake into fuel or energy for the body.

The job of the pancreas is to determine the amount of insulin to produce that is sufficient to regulate the infusion of blood glucose, taken out of the blood stream, into our organs for immediate use, or for storage for future use. Of special importance is the speed at which our bodies get hold of the sugars, in particular, glucose. Insulin unlocks the cells and lets the sugar in. Diabetics have the problem of inadequate glucose management; the sugars remain in useless circulation in the blood stream.

In essence, glucose enters the blood stream, and two things happen simultaneously: blood sugar soars, and insulin, released by the pancreas, also spikes. This spiking has the potential for numerous harmful health issues.

Author Gary Scheiner (2011), who is a certified diabetes educator and person living with diabetes, illustrates the problem as follows:

After meal ["postprandial"] spikes are temporary high blood glucose levels that occur soon after eating.

It is normal for the level of glucose in the blood to rise a small amount after eating, even in people who do not have diabetes. However, if the rise is too high, it can affect your quality of life today and contribute to serious health problems down the road

The obesity problem emerges when there is excess sugar. The relevant scientific explanations relating to the role of insulin, the pancreas, and the matter of sugar spikes are presented in the next chapter.

Starch and sugar must remain in focus, and if you are overweight, you need to beware of various foods to avoid or to be consumed with caution. These include wheat products, flour, rice (including brown rice), cereal types, sugary cereal bars, corn, popcorn, and peas. The reader will be reminded of this simple fact many times throughout this book.

Also, eating sugary foods—that is, starches and carbohydrates—will bring on a kind of double spike. For example, the spikes referred to earlier are higher when a person consumes sweet tea, coffee, smoothies, and beverages with high-sugar content; you can feel it—the rush.

Body fat affects insulin sensitivity across a broad range of conditions. Concern for long-term health also requires the individual with weight management issues to remember that the risk for diabetes and insulin resistance increases as your personal body fat increases, all the way from being very lean to a condition regarded as very obese. A condition of progressing defective insulin secretion management and a rising level of insulin resistance facilitate conditions for the transition from obesity to diabetes. It causes the body to produce more insulin, leading to increased hunger, higher blood pressure, and increased weight gain.

This complex process concerning the pancreas, insulin, and other hormones, especially as they relate to blood sugar control, are presented in the next chapter.

THREE B'S: BREAD, BEER, AND BELLY FAT

I do not believe that I am far off mark if I express the point of view that fat in the midsection or belly is perhaps the hardest to reduce and the one which very often is most evident in obese persons. I am deliberately including a short commentary on the belly-fat image which, regardless of the cause, tends to be referred to by the names indicated in the subtitle above.

Wheat Products: Bread and the "Wheat Belly"

The term "wheat belly" originated from Dr William Davis (2011), author of the book by the same name. He brought to the forefront information on the dramatic impact wheat has on our waistline and our general health. Davis invites his readers to "peer inside" the contents of the grain; he references a multigrain bread advertisement. In his words: "Regardless of shape, color, fibre content, organic or not [wheat] potentially does odd things to humans." (2011)

The starches in wheat are composed of complex carbohydrates. The actual composition is about 75% amylopectin and 25% amylose. Both are digested within the gastrointestinal tract (alimentary canal) and converted to glucose; the process described earlier. You cannot forget: all roads lead to glucose; however, while digestion of the latter is less efficient and some of it reaches the colon in an undigested form, amylopectin converts to glucose rapidly, enters the blood stream, and is mainly responsible for the spike in blood sugar arising from the consumption of wheat products.

Three types of amylopectin exist in various carbohydrate foods, and they are not equal in digestibility. Amylopectin B is found in bananas, potatoes, and is somewhat resistant to digestion. Amylopectin C is found in beans and is the least digestible. In managing obesity, it is amylopectin

A, the kind found in wheat, that is our greatest concern; it is the most digestible form. It is considered a kind of "super carbohydrate," highly digestible and more efficiently converted to blood sugar than almost all the other carbohydrate foods, regardless of whether they are classified as simple or complex.

Let's look at the implications:

> The complex carbohydrates of wheat products, on a gram for gram basis, are no better than, and are often worse than, even simple carbohydrates such as sugar... Whole wheat bread increases blood sugar to a higher level than sucrose... Eating two slices of whole wheat bread is really little different, and often worse, than drinking a can of sugar-sweetened soda or eating a candy bar. [William Davis, 2011]

Consuming a slice of white bread has been approximated to being equivalent to eating a tablespoon of sugar straight from the bowl. It appears to be a waste of time making much fuss about consuming white or multigrain bread. The point of view is that heavily processed wheat in any form, and even wheat in general, is among the worst food items to be consumed by the individual wanting to get rid of unwanted body fat.

It is further advised not to be fooled by the "brown" colour since sneaky manufacturers simply add food colouring to give the healthier look with a whole-wheat appearance.

The point of interest here is that wheat products elevate blood sugar levels much more efficiently than virtually any other carbohydrate. The accompanying insulin spikes facilitate the entry of glucose into the cells of the body with the resulting increase in fat deposit.

One can think of:

> Two slices of bread = more glucose into the blood stream = more insulin spike = more fat deposit.

Call it a "GIF" effect when all three soar: glucose, insulin, and fat deposit. Davis (2011) sums up the wheat belly phenomenon:

Trigger high blood sugars repeatedly and/or over sustained periods, and more fat accumulation results. The consequences of glucose-insulin-fat deposition are especially in the abdomen—resulting in yes, "Wheat-belly." The bigger your wheat belly, the poorer your response to insulin in blood sugar levels and fat storage, since the deep visceral fat of the wheat belly is associated with poor responsiveness; "resistance" to insulin, demanding higher and higher insulin levels, a situation that cultivates diabetes. Moreover, the bigger the wheat belly in males, the more estrogen is produced by fat tissue and the larger the breasts. The bigger your wheat belly, the more inflammatory responses that are triggered: heart disease and cancer.

It would seem advisable that excessive consumption of a western style diet signals significant waist expansion. Good advice for the obese struggler may well be to say goodbye to wheat products i.e. elimination under extreme conditions if the uncomfortable "wheat belly" is to be avoided.

There is interesting additional information on the bread effect. Preparation of bread and pasta with exactly the same ingredients still leads to twice the blood sugar spike from bread and three times the insulin release compared to consuming the same amount of carbs in noodle form. The explanation provided for the difference in the spike is worth remembering. The flour used for making white bread is already stripped of both bran and fibre, and I have already explained the disadvantages of fibre stripping in processed foods. Then the baking process in making bread puffs it up (light, airy slices), and it becomes filled with tiny bubbles allowing digestive enzymes easy access to more surface area, facilitating more rapid digestion of starch into sugars.

Both Davis [2011] and Greger[2019] indicate that the nature of pasta makes it somewhat less effective in popping up blood suga.r levels

This information helps us to understand why bread, in particular white bread, is a forbidden item in meeting the obesity challenge right on! If your obesity problem is serious, take heed: ELIMINATE wheat products. Davis [2011] tells us: " for the most bang for your buck, eliminating wheat is the easiest and most effective step you can take to safeguard your health and trim your waistline". Ratnesar's [1997] article "Against The Grain" focused on the then popular theory relating to "the zone" which emphasized reduced carbohydrate consumption. Meal composition approximated only 40% of calories from carbohydrates and bread was the villain as demonstrated by the sayings: "eat the butter, hold the bread"; also "If all the bread left the face of the earth we'd have a much healthier planet".

Beer: The "Other" Belly Fat

With a continued focus on deep visceral fat of the midsection, we get to know this other belly reference, the "beer belly." The type of sugar in beer is maltose, referred to as the "king" of all sugars, and has a higher glycemic index than white bread; clearly, too much beer consumption places the drinker on the highway to visceral belly fat.

ADDED SUGARS AND OTHER POPULAR SWEETENING FOOD PRODUCTS

Dealing with obesity requires first-response activity with respect to knowing and understanding carbohydrates, starches, and sugars, especially glucose. However, a sustained effort aimed at managing obesity necessitates an awareness of the hidden enemies to success in a range of food items used for sweetening consumable products.

We will learn about added sugars; they are very dangerous and are everywhere.

High-Fructose Corn Syrup

High-fructose corn syrup (HFCS) is a corn-based sweetener used extensively over the past four decades to replace sucrose as the primary sweetener in processed food products, largely because of cost savings. It is a major inclusion in what is called "added sugars"; this group includes sweetening ingredients such as brown sugar, molasses, honey, cane juice, and nectars (fruit, agave), all of which are added to various products classified as processed foods.

HFCS is supposedly 20 times sweeter than sugar and 8 times more addictive than cocaine.

You cannot win the battle in obesity management without being aware of and avoiding HFCS; it has been labeled as the number one enemy in weight management. It is composed of two smaller sugar molecules, glucose and fructose. The fructose portion, "added surreptitiously to processed foods", has been referred to as "a chronic poison" by Lustwig, an endocrinologist at the University of California. [Gorman,2020]. It frequently appears as added sugar and is the "primary cause of metabolic syndrome", a condition discussed in Chapter 6.

In a later chapter, information is provided on what are referred to as the "appetite hormones," ghrelin and leptin. HFCS confuses ghrelin and interrupts leptin, which is responsible for signalling hunger; the resulting brain messaging is incorrect and leads to eating more (Colbert, 2021).

In the standard American diet, it is estimated that these added sugars from all sources can represent as much as 16% of calorie intake, a whopping 300 to 400 calories, and equivalent to about 21 teaspoons of sugar on a daily basis. This means that if you are engaged in the battle of the bulge, you need to be on red alert in watching for hidden sugars.

Honey

There seem to be differing opinions on the use of honey in the battle of the bulge.

It is indicated that its use as a sugar substitute ought to be positive on the basis of animal studies with respect to reducing weight gain and adiposity (fatness). It may improve blood sugar control (Vaccariello, 2012).

It is reported, however, that metabolically, honey has been found to have the same effects as table sugar and high-fructose corn syrup (Greger, 2019).

Maple Syrup

Research is increasingly indicating possible beneficial effects of pure maple syrup, especially Canadian maple syrup, as a sweetener. It carries approximately one third the calories compared to sucrose (pure table sugar); reportedly has some 63 polyphenols, some of them having similar antioxidant benefits to the compounds found in berries, flax seed, red wine, and tea; and each quarter cup provides the recommended daily amount of manganese. Canada' s pure syrup is regarded as having unique chemistry and natural compounds such as point to potential health benefits, including improved sensitivity to the blood sugar regulating hormone, insulin. It does not appear to bring on the same insulin spike as other sugars. Already, I see that maple sugar is being recommended together with raw honey and coconut sugar as healthy alternatives or sugar swaps. Coconut sugar, made from coconut blossom nectar, is 35% less likely to cause blood glucose spikes compared to table sugar. Australian researchers also indicate 400 times more energising potassium.

From my personal experience, when used as a sweetener in moderate amounts, I definitely do not feel the same rush of sugar in my body compared to ordinary sugar or even honey.

Some caution is suggested based on individual research reports, given indications of specific industrial interests financing in some instances. The consensus appears to be that any definitive conclusions on maple syrup must be guided by cumulative additional, creditable research data.

Artificial Sweeteners

Numerous scientific studies have shown that the consumption of added sugars is accompanied by negative effects on human health, especially as it relates to weight gain. In fact, Greger (2019) refers to numerous research studies which have concluded that considering the rapid weight gain that occurs after an increased intake of sugars, it is reasonable to advise individuals on the need for reduced consumption of the substance.

One sweetener, referred to as the "top doc's go-to sweetener" is allulose (*Women's World,* 2023); it is being recommended in facilitating the Keto process with successful weight control; zero carb sugar and zero calories, "slims like magic." It is a natural sugar found in foods such as figs and raisins. The claim is that allulose does not lead to blood sugar issues. Instead, it triggers sugar to burn better and faster and improves insulin sensitivity basically healing damage done by other sweeteners. An additional claim is that allulose boasts a tummy-flattening hormone called adiponectin and that its use has led to shrinking of the waist 1,135% faster compared to persons using Splenda, another very popular sweetener that will be discussed in more detail later in the book.

Studies on the consumption of artificial sweeteners, especially in diet drinks, have also shown a resulting increase in body weight and abdominal fat over time. Sucralose which occurs in Splenda leads to significantly higher blood sugar and insulin spikes. It must also be noted that there is a reported correlation between the adverse effects resulting from the use of as many such noncaloric sweeteners and very pronounced changes in the gut microbiome within a short period of time when used daily.

Yacon Products

Yacon syrup is a frequently mentioned sweetener and the exceptional case where prebiotics have proven effective as an alternative sweetener. It has even been referred to as the next superfood.

Yacon syrup is a natural sweetening agent extracted from tuberous roots of a vegetable plant indigenous to the Andes, apparently historically used by the Incas of Peru. It is referred to as being with "few calories and low sugar"; 1 teaspoon containing only 7 calories (about half the calories of sugar), 3.7 grams of carbs, and 2.3 grams of sugars. One of the major advantages is its high content of insoluble fibres and sugars that cannot be digested. It is one half as sweet as honey and with only one third the calories.

Health claims include it being a gut-healthy alternative to natural, processed sweeteners (like agave) and also artificial sweeteners, such as aspartame, saccharin, and sucralose. Unlike many of these alternatives which generate concern for damaging gut health, it is reported to contribute to gut health by feeding the good bacteria. The explanation regarding its effectiveness as a prebiotic relates to most of its sugars being present as fructans which are indigestible in a general sense while being welcome by friendly gut flora. There is an indication, however, that excess usage can lead to problems related to bloating, diarrhoea, and flatulence.

FURTHER COMMENTARY ON SUGAR

Getting public and political support for limiting sugar intake as a dietary goal has not been easy. "Big Sugar" (the international sugar industry) has traditionally been a powerful and influential lobby, and reportedly, threats against sugar activism. The findings of related science have not been easy to withstand.

The essence of concern is the limitation on intake of added sugars. There is considerable data demonstrating the negative effects of added sugar on metabolism within the body, including the gaining of excess weight. There is general agreement that sugars contribute to obesity and that a reduction in sugar consumption is a matter of top priority in any weight loss programme. The sugar effect on weight management is agreed for both adults and children.

Sugar, however, is proven to have a kind of pleasure-generating effect which promotes overeating, even somewhat related to addiction. An acquired habit of sweet things is not easily broken.

One estimate is that average human consumption within the US is about 50 pounds annually or the equivalent of 17 teaspoons of added sugar daily. Another estimate suggests 152 pounds annually, the equivalent of 3 pounds [6 cups] in a single week. Australian data suggests intake of 60 grams of added sugar (14 teaspoons of white sugar) per day, way off the WHO recommendations of 6 teaspoons for women and 9 for men. The Canadian government recommends 50 grams (12 teaspoons) of added sugar per day; this is in the context of not more than 10% of total daily calorie intake of added sugars.

SUMMARY

This chapter represents a key turning point in the presentation of information relating to obesity. The reader commences the journey at the routine intake of food, the quality of the material chosen by the individual for consumption, and the complex processes involved to achieve energy production for sustaining human life.

Basic food types are briefly discussed; however, wheat products and sugar are highlighted for their role in the struggle faced by any individual confronted with issues of excess body fat and the more extreme condition of obesity.

The chapter introduces the next three which cover the complexities relating to variation in dietary patterns together with the significance of gut bacteria. Special attention is also given to the major role of insulin and issues relating to resistance encountered in the process of complete digestion of food travelling through the human gut.

CHAPTER 5
DIGESTIVE ENZYMES AND GASTROINTESTINAL HEALTH: INTOLERANCE, RESISTANCE, SENSITIVITY, AND MCTS

THIS CHAPTER REPRESENTS a major presentation on matters relating to gastrointestinal health as they impact our core concerns for excess fat and obesity. Gastrointestinal problems affecting obesity relate to abdominal bloating, constipation, impaired nutrient absorption, and excessive weight gain, among other issues. Compared to material presented in all other chapters, the major concepts discussed in this chapter relate to the key words: intolerance, resistance, and sensitivity—all pointing to negative issues in the digestive process.

The previous chapters covered the major issues relating to human nutrition, consumption, and digestion of starches and sugars. The focus has been on the digestive process: why we eat, the main products we consume, and core issues related to inadequate blood sugar control as food passes through the alimentary canal, aka the gastrointestinal (GI) tract. The GI tract is a series of hollow organs joined in a long, twisting tube from the mouth to the anus…the hollow organs that make up the GI tract are the mouth, oesophagus, stomach, small intestine, large intestine, and anus.

The reader is now being exposed to some key concepts involving the science relating to the accumulation of excess body fat and ultimately leading to obesity. Some of the facts presented herein may pose a challenge to individual readers. In this regard, the individual with no or very little interest in the hard science of obesity can skip this chapter with the assurance that the core concepts related to obesity management will have been covered in simple language elsewhere.

In this chapter, the emphasis is on the intricacies of what could go wrong in the digestive process. We take a closer look at the complicated happenings which take place when we eat different foods with different inherent qualities, how the body reacts, and the actual process that leaves us with unwanted and excessive fat deposits in the wrong places. We are then better able to understand the "what" and "why" of necessary changes in lifestyle to emerge victorious in the battle of the bulge.

Chapter 4 introduces a simple classification of carbohydrates as different saccharides (mono-, di-, and so forth), all relating to sugar. We also recall that the digestive process aims at producing simple mono-type sugars which can be absorbed into the blood stream. The three dietary monosaccharides directly absorbed into the blood stream during digestion are fructose, glucose, and galactose. Glucose, the well-known source of energy for complex body processes, is the most familiar monosaccharide or sugar.

We have also paid attention to the significance of the special "S" compounds—sugar and its SOB cousin starch—and their relationship within the sugar story.

At this point, I remind the reader of my personal, self-styled categorisation: the 'SOB' in the struggle with excess body fat and obesity. *It is sugar.* If you have an obesity problem, you will never stop being reminded of the necessity to reduce your sugar consumption; *forget this admonition at your own peril.*

Let me emphasise, however, that in the summary analysis the core issue in scientific terms is that of food energy (taken in) compared to the energy expended (going out/burnt out) in physical activity. The excess is stored as fat.

The hormone, insulin, comes under closer scrutiny than before. Together with other enzymes, they impact efficiency in digestion, including the management of blood sugar levels and GI health in general. Besides insulin, three additional enzymes—amylase, lipase, and protease—comprise the critical trio of very important enzymes impacting digestion. Lipase largely relates to fats and oils while protease relates to proteins. The pancreas, which produces insulin, is also the primary producer of amylase which, since it is released within, is also known as salivary amylase.

CARBOHYDRATE INTOLERANCE, INSULIN RESISTANCE, AND OBESITY

In Chapter 4, relating extensively to digestion and fat, the reader would have gained some basic information on the hormone insulin and its role in the management of blood sugar, fat deposits, and the physical condition referred to as obesity.

We now take a deeper look at this hormone, also known as the hormone of calorie prosperity—a signal of abundance.

Besides the digestion of carbohydrates/starches and sugars and their conversion to sugar, additional major food groups include proteins and fats. When consumed, proteins are converted into amino acids and fats into fatty acids.

The abundance referred to above relates to these three end products: simple sugars, fatty acids, and amino acids—the core end products of the digestive process. Insulin has a major responsibility to take care of the digestion bounty or abundance—that is, the moving or distribution and storage of each of the three end products. It cannot be over emphasised that increased insulin has as its main function sugar distribution in the process of lowering blood sugar to keep blood sugar stable.

The reader is now being provided with information within the context of what I have called "nutritional resistance." The explanation leans heavily on faulty metabolic processes leading to quite serious conditions, all within the context of ill health in the human body. As indicated earlier, sugar remains at the centre of the discussion. We take a close up look at important complications which may arise, especially as they relate to obesity and other health issues.

By whatever categorisation, either of the two "S" words (sugar and starch) or carbs, the human body will attempt to take the conversion all the way to glucose, the simplest sugar, to burn it as a source of fuel. As glucose enters the blood stream, the pancreas releases insulin which helps the glucose in the blood enter muscle, fat, and liver cells to be used for energy or stored for later use. Under normal conditions, the pancreas terminates this action at an appropriate time.

Whenever there is a shortage of the required enzyme to break down or digest the complex carbohydrate to simple sugar, more complex polysaccharides are left behind in the digestive system. The result is elevated blood sugar, and the pancreas works overtime given that the fat, muscle, and liver cells rebel and do not have the normal response expected. The result is elevated blood sugar (hyperglycaemia). The remaining sugars are fermented by the bacteria normally present in the large intestine and in the abdomen, and the ensuing range of effects include cramping, bloating or abdominal distension, flatulence, diarrhoea, and abdominal pain. The severity of the symptoms depends on the extent of the enzyme deficiency. The distress can be felt about 30 minutes to an hour after eating or drinking foods containing the offending sugar.

In essence, the insulin-glucose balancing response described in the previous chapter goes out of whack. Blood sugar levels rise particularly high, even temporarily. While about 40% of consumed carbohydrates are converted to fat in a normal person, the figure becomes 50%–60% with the carbohydrate intolerance or insulin resistance (IR) condition.

Two concepts given special attention are commonly referred to as carbohydrate intolerance (CI) and insulin sensitivity (IS). Different terminology but it all relates to the core of the struggle with serious obesity and weight management problems. CI, IS, and IR are terms which are used interchangeably. Insulin resistance means that the body cells have become resistant to the insulin produced by the pancreas.

Understandably, the various terms used in the literature to essentially reference the same condition has led to CI being referred to as "controversial and confusing." The result of a prolonged CI condition is a worsening roll-over situation towards intolerance. Insulin remains front and centre of the explanation.

One may also encounter the term "gastrointestinal (GI) intolerance." The fact to remember is that an excess intake of carbs or deficiency in the metabolism will result in weight gain. Ultimately, the deteriorating health situation comes under the umbrella of "metabolic syndrome," in essence, a cluster of conditions including the negative health conditions listed above together with the likelihood of a stroke.

Remember that insulin has two controlling responsibilities. Firstly, it controls or regulates blood sugar levels by facilitating storage of *excess* glucose as fat; however, if you're obese , keep in mind that insulin also does a double whammy with respect to fat in our bodies: it can also inhibit the breakdown of fat by a process known as lipolysis; in reality, a breaking up by hydrolysis of the bonds in the tryglycerides. The resulting products are mobilised for stored energy, such as during fasting and exercise. Put simply, insulin can make you fat by interfering with this process.

There is an additional role allotted to insulin: storage, which now looms large in the digestive process when the body cells have sufficient energy. Besides muscle and liver storage of excess sugar (glucose) in the form of glycogen, there is an additional dimension with fat cells also being encouraged to take up glucose and fatty acids to facilitate additional storage.

It is the need for storage of the excess undigested carbohydrates and excess sugars that takes us to the state of obesity. Storage of excess sugar as glycogen in the liver and muscles is limited but there is greater capacity to store the excess carbs, if not burnt off, as body fat in prominent places.

The body can only carry a limited amount of carbs (excess sugar), about 500 grams, as glycogen in muscle and liver cells, equivalent to about 2000 calories of energy. In comparison, a more abundant source of storage is body fat, about 20 times more abundant; this carb or fat tank can accommodate about 40,000 calories.

What makes the problem worse is the fact that as insulin levels rise, it slows considerably the normal preferred metabolic process of burning fat for fuel while at the same time pursuing its food storage function; a kind of double responsibility facilitating both fat deposit and storage at the same time. That's why the general proposition is that as long as the diet is high in carbohydrates, the body has a lower likelihood of burning its own fat for fuel, making weight loss difficult. This is a significant point of outcome determination in the battle against obesity.

Ultimately, we arrive at the juncture of metabolic syndrome (aka syndrome X), representing the end stage where host of related diseases can be encountered, including cancer, heart disease, and the onset of diabetes. The condition of metabolic syndrome signals a "cluster" of risk factors very specific to cardiovascular disease; they include abdominal obesity and high blood pressure.

Reportedly, IR is being linked to increased risk of some cancers, Alzheimer's disease, mental health disorders, and other chronic conditions.

High blood glucose levels tend to lead to early onset of kidney disease and eye retina issues in persons affected with type I diabetes. In type 1 diabetes, the autoimmune system mistakenly kills the body's beta cells which produce insulin. In type 2 diabetes, the body either does not produce enough insulin or cannot use it properly. Individuals affected by type 2 diabetes carry a risk factor for cardiovascular problems. Almost half a billion people worldwide live with type 1 or type 2 diabetes. It is expected that numbers will soar in coming years due primarily to rising rates of obesity. Indications are that while the disease is no longer imminently fatal, it still kills approximately 1.6 million people every year.

Apart from warding off diabetes, managed blood sugar cuts the odds of heart attack, stroke, and dementia by up to 48%. Also, the risk of severe COVID complications drops by about 78%. It is reported that vitamin D plays an important role in the adequate production and regulation of insulin. Low levels are associated with a 40% greater likelihood of developing diabetes. Supplemental daily intake of as much as 2,000 IU has been recommended for optimal health.

Insulin levels at either extreme, too high or too low, are dangerous and damaging to the body. Excessive insulin with intended blood sugar control capability out of whack means that the individual becomes incapable of managing appetite and related food intake.

Food consumption, usually in the form of carbs, is excessive; scrambled brain messages mean blockage of the normal fat burning process. This double-whammy effect is equivalent to programming the body for fat storage, the very opposite effect of what is intended for reducing obesity.

The combination of a reduced insulin effect and faster food movement means that food is not digested fully prior to progressing through the GI tract. The result can be that blood glucose levels rise quite high too soon after eating. In addition, the poorly digested food comes into contact down the road with bacteria in the small intestine and the inadequately or maldigested macronutrients are fermented with a release of gases into the digestive tract and a noticeable buildup of gas.

Development of the conditions described so far means that an individual can face what is known as the "insulin obesity cycle." Obesity kick starts the cycle, leading to insulin resistance and elevated insulin levels then lead to more obesity. For any individual struggling with an obesity problem, a prevailing insulin resistant condition negatively affects all initiatives aimed at fat reduction. Up to 45% of the U.S. population, and similar approximate numbers in other countries, are reported to have insulin resistance. It is also of interest to note that gender appears to show some significant difference in the ability to process carbohydrates. Apparently, obese men are more carbohydrate intolerant than obese women, do not process carbohydrates as efficiently, and are also generally less fit than their female counterparts. Studies also show that more than 70% of obese women are insulin resistant; this rises to 80% if type 2 diabetes is involved (*Women's World*, 2021; Pope).

Our concern with obesity forces us to keep in mind that we cannot focus only on long-term complications. There are serious negative effects on the quality of life anytime blood glucose spikes, even temporarily. Scheiner (2019) reminds us that

> Energy decreases, brain function falters, physical and athletic abilities become diminished and moods become altered... The effects of a bout of post-meal high blood glucose do not go away immediately when blood glucose returns to normal. Each episode... can alter the way certain genes function, resulting in the production of harmful chemicals called free

radicals which cause inflammation and damage to the linings of the blood vessels for hours, if not days.

The worsening condition is known in the medical community as carbohydrate disturbance or hyperinsulinism. It signals more serious conditions such as hypertension, triglyceride levels are elevated together with LDL "bad" cholesterol; HDL "good' cholesterol levels are lowered and body fat deposit increases.

A SPECIAL NOTE: ROLE OF THE LIVER IN OBESITY MANAGEMENT

The liver is the second largest organ in the body after the skin. It is also referred to as a gland. Over 500 functions are indicated, and it holds about 13% of the body's total blood volume. As an organ, it executes chemical reactions; as a gland, it secretes chemicals to be used by other parts of the body.

One of the main functions of the liver is the removal of toxins; oxidation is involved and burnt toxins are removed as bile or urine. The removal of toxins provides numerous benefits, including improved weight management and reduced bloating. The liver is involved in apparently every daily activity of the human body: taking a shower, eating a bagel, drinking a glass of wine, taking your daily prescription. It is the "designated detoxifier" with respect to inspecting intakes into the body and processing and ridding the body of toxic or harmful poisons (James, 2023).

Inefficiency leads to toxin accumulation and hormonal imbalance, both of which lead to stubborn weight gain. When the liver is unable to neutralise or detoxify destructive chemicals that enter the body, they go into storage in fat tissue. Be aware of the "fatty liver" aka "non-alcoholic fatty liver disease," which occurs when the liver is filled with fat and becomes sluggish. The resulting slowing of hormone metabolism leads to hormone imbalance IR. Obese and overweight persons exhibiting IR are more likely to develop fatty liver disease. IR is at the heart of the fundamental problem in obesity and the closely related health defects of heart disease and type 2 diabetes.

Moving out extra toxins from the body by extra flushing, balanced nutrition, and fibre helps to support the body's detox system. The following statement by James (2023) is a summary reminder of an important health issue related to the obesity problem:

> …if you are tired, sluggish and putting on weight, then your body, or more specifically your liver, might be burdened by an excess of toxins that directly prevent it from metabolising nutrients and fats properly. This problem can not only make you constantly tired and overweight, but it can lead to more serious issues such as gallbladder attacks, thyroid problems and more.

The liver has an important role in keeping a host of bodily functions in check; poor maintenance leads to the problems already indicated. It dumps toxins into the gall bladder. The gallbladder stores bile which helps digest fats in the small intestine; large amounts of bile back up and the liver becomes congested. Impeded bile flow means storage rather than a breakdown of fats and definitely a reduction in metabolism.

An effective detox programme means toxin elimination; when complemented with essential vitamins, detox facilitates improved weight management and increased energy/vitality.

ADDITIONAL SIGNIFICANT HORMONES IN THE CONTROL OF OBESITY: LEPTIN AND GHRELIN

The hypothalamus, an important part of the brain, is known as the master regulator of metabolism and plays a significant role in the regulation of food consumption and weight management issues. It also controls vital body functions, blood circulation, metabolism, stress, emotional expression, sexual behaviour and memory, body temperature, and body fat, the latter by causing increased consumption when one gets too and less when too fat.

Two hormones mentioned earlier, leptin and ghrelin, signal fullness or hunger to the brain. Ghrelin stimulates and leptin inhibits appetite.

Excessive insulin reportedly scrambles their signalling capability; false messages are received.

Leptin, a hormone released from fat cells in adipose (fat) tissue, signals to the hypothalamus, playing a crucial role in food intake over the long-term. Its release is somewhat controlled by insulin. It is our "satiety centre," carefully controlling our appetites and regulates the body's response to signals from the stomach indicating that it is full.

The effective functioning or level of release into our blood stream is directly related to the level of fat on our bodies. When blood leptin levels get too high our appetite is down regulated (Greger, 2019, p. 103). Losing weight means that levels of the hormone fall and this in turn stimulates appetite and food intake. This signalling mechanism works well in lean persons but the efficiency declines with overweight individuals. In general, it does help with maintaining "normal" weight and can create difficulty in weight loss for the typical dieter.

When the hypothalamus is damaged, there is interference with the normal feedback loop within the brain and it can no longer respond adequately to the signals on blood leptin levels intended to affect weight control. This creates a condition in which overweight individuals produce enough leptin secreted by their excess fat, but the leptin control influence is blunted since the hypothalamus is resistant. There is damage to the leptin-hypothalamus circuit and the result is hypothalamic obesity due to "hypothalamic dysfunction" (Greger, 2019, p. 107).

AMYLIN

The effect of salivary amylase, mentioned earlier, in the mouth represents the so-called first step in the chemical digestion of food. This knowledge reminds us of the importance of taking time to chew food thoroughly in the mouth. Failure to do so implies inadequate food breakdown and a deficiency in the ultimate liberation of nutrients to be made available for later absorption in the digestive process.

Together with insulin, amylase also makes an important contribution in the control of blood sugar, especially regarding the consumption of carbohydrates and sugars. Any deficiency in this regard can result in the individual encountering serious health problems.

Amylase is responsible for controlling the speed of food as it moves from the stomach towards the small intestine where nutrients are absorbed and allowed to flow into the blood stream.

Insulin takes about 15 minutes or less to swing into action following food intake; about 60–90 minutes to peak or reach maximum effectiveness and about 4 hours or more to finish working. When amylin is either produced in insufficient amounts or not at all, its "traffic cop" effect is missing. Food movement from the stomach to the intestine is not slowed the way it should be and is, therefore, digested even faster than usual.

HUMAN GROWTH HORMONE: HORMONE RESCUE

Human growth hormone (HGH) is normally produced by the pituitary gland. "Hormone Rescue," a powerful visual headline appears in a recent article in Woman's World, March 21, 2022. It references "slimming power of an often-forgotten hormone… HGH… lose up to 40 lbs in 30 days!" and indicates treatment activity involving medical training at a very prestigious U.S. university. The reverse of HGH decline with age is indicated, as much as 50% by age 50. The accompanying strategies include keto type dieting. A high intake of eggs, fish, and beef are associated with increased quantities of HGH as is an exercise regime and controlled eating pattern. HGH is an active ingredient in many prescription drugs and is widely available.

Indications are that individuals have tried HGH pills, powders, and injections; however, there does not seem to be any adequate research findings to justify increasing HGH intake, more so by these artificial methods to achieve effective weight management.

THE MCT STORY: A SPECIAL KIND OF FAT

In the pursuit of ways and means to tackle excess fat storage in the human body, researchers have paid special attention to a group of complex carbohydrates known as medium-chain triglycerides (MCTs), commercially available as various brands of MCT oil. They represent a type of fat that is more easily digested and more rapidly metabolised for energy than other types of fats.

References to MCT turn up everywhere in the dialogue on weight reduction with particular reference as to how to achieve success in the "burning off" of stubborn fat from the obese torso.

The use of MCT oil is a major aspect of the highly commercialised Keto diet discussed in the next chapter.

MCT Oil and the Insulin Challenge

Before any transformation takes place, fats are naturally found in foods in a triglyceride formulation. When digested, fatty acids are let loose and are ready for absorption within the small intestine. The structure of fatty acids—that is, the number of carbon atoms or length of the carbon chain in each structure—determines how the fatty acid is absorbed and used by the body.

MCT oil falls within the subgroup of medium-length or medium-chain triglycerides which carry a lower number of atoms. They are shorter in length and have the unique ability to quickly cross over from the digestive system into blood circulation. This means rapid movement or absorption into the liver, where with minimal action, they are readily availability for conversion to energy.

For clarification, MCTs have between 6 and 8 carbon molecules compared to 10–12 in long-chain triglycerides (LCTs). The LCTs remain in the body longer and are more likely to be stored as fat, excessive quantities of which we associate with obesity.

MCT oil provides the special group of fats which convert to ketones, a different and new preferred major source of energy. It becomes an alternative to glycogen derived from carbohydrates and stored by the liver. The alternative state of energy conversion and provision is called ketosis.

Pure MCT is difficult to find. Most commercial products are a mixture of coconut and palm oil. Coconut is very frequently referenced as a source of MCT, perhaps the best source, seeing that it contains the highest concentration of MCT (55%) in any food. It is also harvested from palm oil, a supposedly cheaper source but not as good. Commercial brands boast of having varying percentages of pure MCT. Coconut oil also has other fats which slow down absorption. If used for cooking, it is advisable to use a MCT supplement which carries a more concentrated form of MCTs.

A visit to a good health supplement store can be overwhelming with the different choices for MCT oil; this suggests some caution in determining which one to purchase. Be aware that there are four different types of MCT oil, knowledge of which may assist in purchasing choices. The four different medium-chain fatty acids in MCT oils are caproic acid (C6), caprylic acid (C8), capric acid (C100, and lauric acid (C12).

Reported conclusions from experimental trials with MCT vary considerably. In general, however, MCT oil is supposed to both increase calorie burn and decrease calorie consumption. Reported results include demonstrated fat loss of about 1.83 pounds per week, a potential 24-pound loss of pure fat in a year. In comparison with olive oil, users of MCT oil were found to lose more than 2.5 times as much fat and also significantly more upper body fat compared to the group using olive oil. Reportedly, higher application doses have been shown to help women burn an extra 190 calories per day. Anticipated additional 40% weight loss was projected for individuals using a high dosage in one experiment when compared to non-participants.

It has been suggested that MCT can be used instead of olive oil for dietary purposes, such as in salad dressings, marinades, or even smoothies. There is also a product produced by blending MCT oil and coconut oil for individuals who experience stomach disorders when taking undiluted MCT oil ("Heal Your Guy, Lose Your Belly Fat," 2016).

Numerous advertisements tout the advantages of coconut and MCT for ladies whose cultural and geographical circumstances favour more attention to coconut as part of their staple diet and the application of commercial products for improved health and beauty including "increased metabolism and with easier weight loss" [www.menopausenaturalsolutions.com/blog/MCT-and-menopause; https://lk.spaceceylon]

Some authors suggest an inadequacy of research data to make finite conclusions on the efficacy of MCTs. In the interim, however, the additional health benefits touted of MCT supplementation include the following:

1. Enhanced brain function. Indications are that ketones are a more efficient source of energy for the brain compared to glucose and suggest improved mental clarity and focus.

2. Reduced fat storage, given the provision of an instant source of energy; increased thermic (burning) effect on food meaning increased caloric burning with less storage.

3. Especially effective in burning stubborn belly fat.

4. The increased ketone production suppresses the hormone ghrelin which creates the feeling of being hungry.

5. Improved gut health. MCT oil alters the composition of gut bacteria, encouraging the growth of healthy bacteria in the microbiome.

6. When consumed before intense exercise, it reduces lactate build-up in muscles and facilitates greater exercise endurance.

7. Improves insulin sensitivity of persons with type 2 diabetes and assists in the control of blood sugar.

Significance of MCT Oil in Weight Management Initiatives

The keto diet appears to have a global fan base. MCT is a major ingredient in the application of the keto dietary principle; discussed in greater detail in Chapter 7, a focus on selected dietary types. MCT represents that special group of fats which facilitate what is known as the ketogenic transformation.

Keto weight management philosophy emphasises a core dietary choice of low carbohydrates-high fat as the route to successful weight management. In this regard, MCT is declared as being healthier than other saturated fats. Proponents of the diet emphasise keto adaptation (aka "fat adapting") with the metabolic shift in the primary source of energy.

The governing theory is that lower daily carbs intake reduces the use of sugar as a source of energy on the intake side of the equation and shifts the body's metabolic system to burning already stored (accumulated) fat. Later on, after successful body fat reduction, dietary management requires that carbohydrate uptake be dialed back up gradually to meet sustainable daily dietary requirement levels.

SUMMARY

This chapter represents closure of my presentation on the science relating to metabolic processes beyond initial food intake and the circumstances which lead to undesirable health conditions. It provides a foundational explanation of the focal subject of this book: issues related to excessive body fat often rolling over to the more extreme condition which qualifies an individual as being obese.

Blood sugar level issues are dealt with under a host of different scientific names. By whatever name, related hormonal relationships and their impact on personal health need to be understood both for obesity and diabetes-affected individuals; the latter may or may not have a double complication. In any case, post-meal high blood glucose (post-prandial hyperglycemia) is a condition worthy of special attention whenever it surfaces in any individual. Understanding how it all works and the related personal management actions will impact an understanding of the lifestyle changes necessary to deal with obesity.

CHAPTER 6
SELECTED PROMINENT DIET TYPES AS SYSTEMS OF AGGRESSIVE FOOD-INTAKE CONTROL

ONE VERY INTERESTING finding from the research effort in the evolution of this book is the need for caution by individuals who are inclined to pursue one or more commercial diets. Many of these are quite prominent in the media with quite a few offering phenomenal claims for successful weight management. There is an endless array of diets from which to choose. In recent times, there have emerged delivered-to-your-door meal plans.

One publisher indicates that the average advertised testimonial weight loss across 20 different programmes was about 50 pounds (22.7 kg), a number far in excess of what even the programmes' own published trials have shown. Beyond this, regarding success stories used in advertisements, including the use of narratives, the general picture is not convincing with respect to various initiatives aimed at evaluation of commercial claims relating to "guaranteed" weight loss. When researchers actually followed up on some of the people portrayed in the before and after pictures, only about one in four appears to have sustained their success. Most ads made at least one claim that was very likely to be false or, at the very least, lacking adequate substantiation [Greger, 2019]

There are numerous diets. In addition, there are some descriptive control systems not labelled as such but with the same generally intended outcomes. I have provided information on a few selected popular diet types together with brief notations on systems included in the literature on diets. Interest in the details will vary among readers; however, it all relates to persons in search of an effective pattern of food intake management to aid in personal weight control. Some persons, especially older individuals, pursue diets to protect long-term health and to prevent reoccurrence of previously experienced health issues.

THE ATKINS DIET (LOW CARBOHYDRATE, HIGH PROTEIN)

The original core principle of the Atkins diet emphasises an almost non-inclusion of carbohydrates (low carb) and a dependency on proteins; it allows for an almost limitless use of saturated fats (butter, red meat, and so forth). This fits the typical low-carb, ketogenic diet—the very opposite of the low-fat regime also being promoted as gospel at the time the Atkins diet emerged. The combination of low carbs with high saturated fats means that the body turns to burning fat for fuel via the process of ketosis which is considered in greater detail later in the chapter.

Revised versions have surfaced over time, such as the "New Atkins for a New You" which supposedly represents a revolutionized approach to low-carb eating and offers greater flexibility and maintenance in lifestyle. The Atkins website (www.atkins.com) offers many recipes. The revised version allows for intake of larger portions of fibre and is based upon a better understanding of its minimal effect on blood sugar levels. High-fibre veggies are promoted.

An important assumption of the low-carb advocacy was that of reduced insulin levels. Indications are that the decline is very small; however, there is, instead, a notable rise in what is referred to as bad LDL cholesterol levels with serious problems related to impaired artery function and reduced life spans. Opinions vary on the effects of this process which happens to be the lynchpin of some other diets. There are indications of problems for individuals with kidney problems or who are on certain kinds of medications.

THE SOUTH BEACH DIET

The South Beach Diet was developed by Dr. Arthur Agatston, a cardiologist in the southern USA. He states it is neither low fat or low carb but that the focus is on the right carbs and the right fats (right meaning "good") and indicates a possible weight loss of 8–13 pounds within 2 weeks. [[Agatston, 2003]

He comments that the primary failing of many diets promoted is that they are "too complicated and too rigid" and possibly medically sound but hard to maintain in real life, the experts never allowing for human frailty or allowing for accommodation of behavioural slips along the way. He also aims to achieve a diet that is "lively and diverse" with some adaptability to one's personal tastes and habits.

His first two weeks carries some specific pointers:

1. no bread, rice, potatoes, pasta, or baked goods
2. no candy, cake, cookies, ice cream, or sugar
3. no alcohol, beer, or wine of any kind.

The first two weeks accomplishes a major internal change, correcting "the way the body reacts to the very foods that cause overweight" and the physical craving which favouring bad foods will be "switched off" and remain like that so long as the diet is followed. There is a change in the body's response to food.

Some of the banned foods are introduced into the dietary pattern later on in Phase 2, including pasta and bread, but on a limited scale. The individual remains in Phase 2 until the goal for weight loss is reached.

Phase 3 is a modified version of Phase 2 and lasts for life.

Ultimately, the plan supposedly allows for normal-size servings of meat and fish of all types; plenty of vegetables, eggs, cheese, and nuts; salads with real olive oil in the dressing; and three balanced meals per day, enough to satisfy hunger.

The author emphasises a switch from poor eating habits which contribute to a blood chemistry profile dangerously high in cholesterol and triglycerides. There is a focus on cutting out bad (highly processed) carbohydrates from which most of the fibre is removed, encouraging good carbohydrates (fruits, vegetables, and whole grains). The diet permits a range of sources of fats and animal protein including lean beef, pork, veal, and lamb and encourages the use of oily fish types including salmon, tuna, and mackerel. Egg yolk is cited as a source of natural vitamin E, and nuts and low-fat dairy products (cheese, milk, yogurt) are allowed. Mono- and polyunsaturated fats, including olive oil, canola oil, and peanut oil are listed as good fats and encouraged.

THE PALEO DIET (LOW CARBOHYDRATE, HIGH PROTEIN)

The paleo diet is regarded as being very popular, the industry being worth some US$500 million in 2019 based upon products with the word "paleo" included. It is also referred to by other names including Paleolithic, paleo-caveman, and Stone Age. The Paleolithic, aka Old Stone Age, is referred to as a period in prehistory distinguished by the development of stone tools. The major characteristics were the dependency of the inhabitants on their environment. They were typically nomadic with men being hunters and women being gatherers. In essence it is described as mirroring foods eaten during the Paleolithic era, allowing for consumption of those foods that humans ate when they first roamed the planet millions of years ago. Variations in requirements exist, some being predominantly plant-based. There is a little more inclusion of animal products in recent times. It is viewed favourably by the opposition to veganism.

In this diet, processed food is avoided, but vegetables, fruits, nuts, roots, and meat are included. It also excludes dairy products, grains, sugar, legumes, processed oils, salt, alcohol, and coffee.

Reportedly, research evidence suggests advantages for improved health compared to the typical Western diet and some European nutritional guidelines. There is an indication of nutritional deficiencies, including inadequate calcium intake and side effects such as weakness, diarrhoea, and headaches. Some research analysis has shown negative effects on cholesterol levels.

THE KETO DIET (HIGH FAT, LOW CARBOHYDRATE)

The keto diet is very popular; information bombards the senses on almost every available platform or website which caters to human health. The word "keto" dominates diet plans, pills, coffee, and all kinds of pharmaceuticals and snacks—all sold as a miracle way to tackle obesity successfully. The global keto market is estimated at $10.2 billion and is projected to reach $15.27 billion by 2027 (Reed, 2023).

It has received considerable prominence in the management of weight loss and the treatment of type 2 diabetes. The high-fat, low-carbohydrate formula has been extensively commercialized and keto products abound globally. While other low carbohydrate diets focus on protein, the keto diet focuses on fat which may provide as much as 90% of daily calories.

Limited unsaturated fats, including nuts (almonds, walnuts), avocados, and olive oil, are allowed. However, saturated fats from oils (coconut and palm oils [major sources of MCT]), lard, butter, and cocoa butter are encouraged. The basic dietary pattern is one of eating foods rich in fats and with moderate intake of protein and very low intake of carbohydrates.

Carbohydrate deprivation is vital: less than 20–50 grams per day. The body is literally starved for its preferred fuel, glucose. Our body chemistry changes; there is a run on the burning of body fat for energy thereby reducing available fat for storage and consequently less fat to deposit such as would lead to an accompanying weight gain and the resulting obesity. It also emphasises that restricted carbohydrate intake means less insulin secretion and less fat storage since more is burnt as an alternative fuel.

The process facilitates a switch from blood sugar to ketones as an alternative primary fuel source for life sustaining activity. These ketones are an alternative to stored glycogen derived from excessive carbohydrate intake. The change in fuel supply heralds the ketogenic state; aka ketosis.

The core recommendations of the keto diet as laid out by prominent author Don Colbert (2017) in his comprehensive publications, including *Keto Zone Diet*, are as follows:

1. The standard keto diet is 70% from fat, 25% from proteins, and 5% from carbs.
2. Fat automatically burns faster.

3. It's necessary to recognise the importance of good bacteria (the fibre in plants being a good source).

4. Good bacteria reverses problems experienced with insulin which is involved in hampering progress with weight loss in about 70% of adults.

5. Important to incorporate lots of keto-friendly veggies in the diet: leafy greens, onions, cruciferous (cauliflower, broccoli, cabbage) veggies, asparagus, mushrooms, asparagus, bell peppers, cucumber, and celery.

6. Go for fibre-rich sources of fat (avocados).

7. Avoid hydrogenated oils, artificial flavours and colours, excess sodium, fat, and refined sugar.

8. Avoid items labelled as "low fat" and "fat free"; they all have added sugars. Beware of the carb related Olean used extensively in products such as potato chips.

9. Watch labels. Sugar is often hidden under various labels, including HFCS, evaporated cane juice solids, fruit juice concentrates, and be cautious of fruits high in sugars.

It is to be noted that quite a few diet types, including paleo, Atkins, and South Beach, have sometimes been placed within the keto-type diet; however, real keto focuses on fat, a must at each meal, not protein, and can reach as much as 90% of the daily calories. The diet is high in saturated fat

While there appears to be considerable conviction that the diet is effective for weight loss, it is important .to note that effective pursuit of the keto programme requires the individual to keep track of blood ketone levels in order to ensure stability within the fat-burning zone. It is reported that some 70% of participants do not undertake this important tracking activity and that almost one half of the individuals cheat on the diet. The top cheating foods include carbs (bread, pasta, and potatoes, including all forms of chips), deserts and sweets, wine and beer, and rice.

Various kinds of criticism have been made of the keto dietary pattern. The keto carbohydrate restriction base theory has been described as faulty with the suggestion that a dietary fat restriction model may be more efficient. The level of saturated fat, given its association with increase in bad

LDL and heart disease, is considered one of the top risks with this diet. There is also a potential risk regarding deficiencies in micronutrients, including selenium, magnesium, phosphorus, and vitamins B and C. Long term efficiency has been questioned and the diet has been referred to as "a medical diet that comes with serious risks" [Harvard Health Publishing, 2020]

MEDITERRANEAN-LABELLED DIETS

The Mediterranean Diet

The Mediterranean diet derives its name from traditional eating habits in the 16 countries bordering the Mediterranean Sea. This means that there is no single standard which applies to all of them, given the variation, even within a single country, of geography, ethnic differences, religion, and culture. However, there are a few well-established staples, including olive oil, high intake of fresh fruit and vegetables, moderate fish and dairy intake, and limited red meat, saturated fats, whole grains, and, of course, wine. There is generally no meat (including fish in some references), eggs, or dairy on a day-to-day basis. The resulting dominance of so-called short-chain fatty acid levels is somewhat comparable to levels seen for vegans.

This diet is essentially a low-carb strategy which reduces glucose overload; it is in short supply and fat becomes an alternative to glucose as a source of fuel for energy. The dieting patterns are based on restricted intake of starchy carbs and an emphasis on veggies combined with fish, poultry, nuts, and olive oil. Restricting carb intake to about 20–40 grams per day in the beginning provides a kickstart in metabolic conversion that taps into fat reserves in the body. This is of particular importance in tackling stubborn serious visceral belly fat usually associated with blood pressure and cholesterol issues and insulin imbalance. The projected effect is loss of water weight together with 6 lb of fat per week and as much as 18 lb in a month.

Some important characteristics of the Mediterranean diet include:

- Processed carbs are replaced by a diet rich in Mediterranean fare, such as grilled chicken or fish

- Unlimited quantities of fish, especially cold-water types such as trout, salmon, sardines, mackerel, tuna, halibut, seabass, herring, and tuna
- Three servings of vegetables (1–1½ cups) daily, including broccoli, cucumbers, mushroom, eggplant, artichokes, leafy greens, bell peppers, and cauliflower
- Virgin or extra virgin oil with meals (2–3 tablespoons)
- Snacks: a handful of nuts is common.

Recent research (January 2023) out of Harvard University draws attention to the positive effect of the presence of polyphenols in blueberries, olives, and red wine, staples of this diet. Increasing the supply of phenols maximises the slimming effect of the Mediterranean diet. When spirulina is added, for example in smoothies, increased fat loss is to be as much as 27% higher (*First for Women*, 2023).

The traditional Mediterranean diet is associated with better cardiovascular health, including a reduction in total cardiovascular disease and reduced rates of ischemic stroke and coronary heart disease. Reportedly, high heart risk individuals who followed this diet supplemented with extra virgin oil or nuts were less likely to succumb to heart attack or stroke or die from heart disease compared to persons merely following a low-fat diet (Harvard Medical School, 2020).

Even though the Mediterranean diet adherents are not completely plant-based all the time, its benefits are somewhat related to the advantages of a plant-based dietary intake.

Dietary Approaches to Stop Hypertension Diet

The Dietary Approach to Stop Hypertension (DASH) Diet is also considered plant-based, reducing saturated fat intake, and gets high marks in the world of diets. It features special measures to restrict sodium and lower blood pressure. It is also recognised as the MIND Diet (Mediterranean-DASH Intervention for Neurodegenerative Delay).

This diet was originally developed at the Rush University Medical Center with a focus on having beneficial effects on hypertension. Later on, its reformulation touted the additional feature of weight loss. It is also reported to have lowered the risk of Alzheimer's by 35% with moderate compliance, and as high as 53% with rigorous adherence.

The simple dietary outline includes some core recommendations which accompany many other proposals for healthy eating. Its quantity and range of nutrients are considerably more than other diets, and it has been referred to as "one of the great breakthroughs in nutrition." A special feature is its inclusion in adequate quantities of the combination of nutrients and fibre, referred to as the "fighting four": fibre, calcium, vitamin D, and omega-3s. Positive weight loss results indicated as much as 8 lb per week.

The designers simply have two categories of specific food types, to be included copiously or to be limited in use. This includes:

- Green leafy vegetables: every day
- Fruit and non-starchy vegetables: 8–10 servings per day
- Whole grains and/or starchy veggies: 3 servings per day
- Nuts: one small serving every day
- Wine: one glass per day
- Beans: every other day
- Berries: at least twice per week, especially blueberries and strawberries
- Poultry: at least twice per week
- Fish: at least once per week
- Low-fat or non-fat (healthy dairy): 2 –3 servings
- Olive oil
- To be limited:
- Red (fatty) meats: fewer than 4 servings per week
- Butter and margarine: less than 1 tablespoon per day
- Cheese: less than 1 serving per week
- Fried and fast food: less than 1 serving per week
- Refined sugars and carbohydrates, including sugar sweet-ened beverages
- Sodium (salt) 2,300 mg per day; when used in excess, it supposedly results in excessive fat storage.

This diet is apparently recommended widely by medical personnel from many prominent institutions. The advocates of the DASH diet clearly recognise its limitation as a strategy for weight loss by itself. When combined with exercise and some reduction in calorie intake, however, the diet has supposedly proved very effective in the reduction of blood pressure and a resulting need for continued medication.

The DASH and MIND diets referred to above represent very much what is indicated as the basic dietary pattern in what Karst (2023) refers to, geographically, as the five Blue Zone locations. These were discovered in 2004 by a team of medical researchers, anthropologists, and epidemiologists in search of locations where people live long, healthy, and happy lives. The locations include Sardinia, Italy; Ikaria, Greece; Nicoya Peninsula, Costa Rica; Seventh Day Adventists in Loma Linda, California; and Okinawa, Japan. The diet comprises 85% of vegetables, fruits, grain, and legumes, and is generally devoid of large portions of meat, sugar, and processed foods. Daily consumption of wine (one to two glasses), coffee, or black tea is indicated. It is emphasised that people in these locations stop eating when they are 80% full; the feeling of being stuffed is avoided. The basic eating pattern is crucial and fits into an intermittent fasting (IF) schedule discussed later in the chapter; a small meal in late afternoon or early evening and nothing else is eaten for the rest of the day. A strong sense of family and community connections are foundational to the Blue Zone lifestyle.

Commentary: Recent research on Mediterranean-Type diets and Parkinson's Disease

Recent research by Apple-Creswell and others at the University of British Columbia with a focus on the MIND diet indicates a positive relationship between healthy Mediterranean-type diets and a lower risk of developing Parkinson's disease. The age of onset of the disease in men adhering to the Greek Mediterranean diet was up to eight years later compared to men adhering to the typical Western-type diet (typically rich in red meat and processed, fried, sweetened and pre-packaged foods). For women on the MIND diet, the onset age was up to 17 years later.

THE MARTHA'S VINEYARD DIET DETOX

The authorship of the Martha's Vineyard diet is Dr. Roni Luz. The regime emphasises simplicity and the use of anti-inflammatory ingredients in achieving the release of a lot of fat. Necessary kitchen utensils equipment include blenders and juicers to make the plan's green drinks, berry smoothies, and creamy soups. The diet's premise is as follows:

- Liquids and purees facilitate immediate entry into the blood stream with instant reduction of inflammation and healing of cells and organs
- Digestive systems weaken with cumulative age and experience increasing difficulty extracting vitamins, minerals, and antioxidants from food. Blended food allows improved absorption of nutrients
- No animal protein means easier nutrient absorption and allows for smaller intake quantities on each occasion.
- Detox facilitates shrinkage of fat cells.

Success of this diet boasts a loss of 21 pounds in 21 days (https://mvdietdetox.com/) or approximately 10 pounds the first week. It is also suggested that the plan can achieve losses of 39 pounds in 21 days. One version of the plan references morning (8 a.m.), afternoon (2 p.m.), and evening (6 p.m.) "sips" of soup of blended recipe items.

THE PRITIKIN PROGRAM'S CALORIE DENSITY SOLUTION

The Pritikin program offers an array of meals, the quality of each one being determined essentially by its calorie density.

Pritikin discards ideas or principles relating to the need for an element of hunger, eating lots of high-protein foods loaded with fat or cholesterol, and the need for an array of low-fat foods, including popcorn and whole grain breakfast cereals. The more recent approach announces new perspectives compared to the old Pritikin recommendations referred to as being "buried"

The calorie density principle allows the individual to "eat as much as you want… as often as you desire and still lose weight." In essence, calorie density is regarded as the story behind weight gain!. It is essentially a low fat and high fibre regimen limiting red meat, alcohol and processed food items

Reference is made to research data that demonstrates "calorie density alone... being... the single most important factor that determines calorie intake, weight loss or weight gain."

A major decision to eat a diet low in calorie density is to fill your stomach and satisfy your tastebuds on as few calories as possible. This strategy seeks to achieve low calorie, high nutrient density.

Three dietary plans are offered with successively lower calorie densities: Better, Better Still, and Best—each level reflecting the meal's quality according to calorie density.

In summary, the programme recommends eating three low-calorie dense meals per day, along with two or three snacks between meals, all of which must also be low in calorie density.

Criticism of the diet has included being boring unpalatable and with a low level of compliance

[The Pritikin Diet Plan Cookbook, 2021 Edition; Overview. Indigo internet site.- www.indigo.ca/en-ca/updated-pritikin-diet-plan cookbook 2021 edition][Pritikin 1988]

THE NOOM WEIGHT CONTROL PROGRAMME

Relatively new with respect to behaviours intended to assure success in weight loss is Noom, a consumer-led digital health company that helps people live healthier and, supposedly, happier lives. It claims to go beyond other weight-loss programs which emphasise the "what" and "why" of what is eaten. It is an approach based on research in psychology and behavioural science; the system recommendations engage the way individuals think and feel about eating, why and how behaviours impact health. [noom.com]

It is a personalized curriculum with a focus on changing long term habits. There is an emphasis on the "WHY" behind one's personal condition. The system explores the reasons for individual personal behaviour. No food item is labeled "bad" or off limit. It emphasises that true weight loss is about so much more than the calories in vs out perspective.

[Noom Team, 2022]

Noom self-describes as "the world's leading behavior change company, disrupting the weight loss and health care industries." It represents the combined power of artificial intelligence, mobile technology, and psychology together with the input of empathy of over 1,000 personal coaches.

According to Noom's website (2023), "Noom Weight is *not* a fad diet or an elimination diet." There is no definitive requirement with respect to cutting carbohydrates or the use of a point system for rewarding the participant. The system infuses a bit of science into the mind of the target subject and claims that participants will learn:

- What triggers you to eat when you're not hungry
- How to overcome emotional and stress eating
- What to do instead of reaching for a snack when you don't feel good
- How incorporate mindfulness while eating
- How to choose foods that pack a powerful nutrition punch (but still keep you feeling full and satisfied)
- How to tell the difference between feeling genuinely hungry and 'head hungry'
- How to manage plateaus (when your weight loss temporarily stalls) (Noom, 2023)

Unlike the typical diet, it does not aim to restrict or deprive a person of their favourite foods or food groups. It aims to help an individual understand and adopt lasting and sustainable personal eating habits which lead to successful weight-loss management, instead of what turns out to be temporary fixes. A major objective in the system is to enable the individual to remain within an effective calorie range, resulting in a feeling of satisfaction within fewer calories. The programme offers calorie counting activity and facilitates group support from "supportive Noomers."

Personal coaching, in part using a phone app, is an important feature and is key to achieving success; it has been referred to as "a dietician in your pocket" or "accountability coaching."

Noom has also developed a virtual diabetes program with its platform already in use by leading pharmaceutical and healthcare companies. There are two well-known offers based upon the Noom approach: Noom Mood for mental health support involved in stress reduction in the workplace and a resulting improved performance affecting absenteeism and productivity, and Noom Weight, which is more of the core programme focussed on weight control; a focus on choices, the "why," and the creation of sustainable habits.

An interesting feature for guidance is the use of a colour scheme which covers a range of food items: from high nutrient/low calorie (green) to low nutrient/high calorie (red). Nothing is forbidden; however, participants are encouraged to eat mostly green and red foods.

GOLO WEIGHT LOSS PROGRAM

The GOLO programme is reportedly designed by medical professionals. There is an indication of some similarity to the Noom programme: no emphasis on calorie counting and with a focus to educate people of all ages. The objective is to achieve long-term lifestyle modification. The admonition is to stop dieting and is presented as a safe alternative to drastic weight-loss initiatives. The advertisement stresses, inter alia, no cutting of food groups, no diet plateau, no isolation, and no hunger cravings.

INTERMITTENT FASTING: A SYSTEM OF AGGRESSIVELY CONTROLLED FOOD INTAKE

Intermittent fasting regimes come with a variety of calorie-intake options. In general, they can be described as dietary patterns in which an individual decides to confine food intake to a particular period during a 24-hour day, over a period of time. In instances of highly restrictive food intake, items may be restricted to water, tea, coffee, and other low-calorie or non-caloric drinks. The diet period may be scheduled so that the individual is asleep for most of the fast period. The result, generally, is a severe restriction on the calories consumed.

Some examples of variation in IF regimes are:
- Eating as much as you want every other day ("alternate days")
- Eating as much as you want during a fixed few hours of each day
- Fasting for 2 days a week or 5 days a month
- Ramadan, the month-long period of fasting by practising Muslims
- Abstention from food and drink from sunrise to sunset.
- Eating one meal a day (OMAD)

Hereunder are some examples of controlled food intake reflecting IF system.

The 16:8 Diet Plan

Eating takes place during a chosen 8-hour period of the day. A decision may be that eating does not go beyond a chosen hour, such as 6 or 7 p.m., and there is a 16-hour non-eating gap between periods which includes sleep time.

The long intermittent periods reduce food intake and blood sugar highs and lows, and sends the body into fat-burning mode (including visceral belly fat), as compared to burning glucose. It is not recommended for persons using insulin, with an eating disorder, or who are pregnant or planning to be. Appetite control, which lowers the effect of the hunger hormone ghrelin, is critical in achieving a reduction of calorie intake; the pattern has been shown to reduce calorie intake by as much as 350 calories per day.

The System 20 Plan

Recently, an IF "System 20" plan was introduced on the famous Dr. Oz television show. The details are also published in his "Best Slim Down Tips" indicated in a list of 20 things doable in 2020 with the objective of losing 20 pounds and enjoying the well-known health benefits of weight control. The focus is on brunch and dinner. Breakfast is skipped, but there is morning coffee with MCT oil. Fast from 7 p.m. to protein brunch at 11 a.m.; eat no added sugars; snack on low-carb snacks; and add 2 table-spoons of apple cider vinegar to lunch or dinner.

One case reported losing 55 pounds in 3 months, "melting 23 inches off her waistline and curing her sleep apnea" (Maxbauer, 2022).

The Mosely and Spencer Plan

Mosley and Spencer express the point of view that IF can have a "revolu-tionary, game changing effect" on human health. Subjecting individuals to cyclical fasting of "feast or famine" leads to an improved metabolic status. They reference research which shows a resulting increased insulin action on whole body glucose uptake and lipolysis on adipose tissue. A simple explanation is that while the body at rest burns a 50:50 mix of carbs and fat, moving into an IF regime leads to a real scarcity of stored glycogen within 12–36 hours after eating ceases. Thereafter, there is a metabolic switch to reliance on stored fat. Keep in mind, therefore, that with respect to a 3-day fasting initiative, the greatest breakdown and burning of fat occurs within that period of 18–24 hours within the 72-hour time span. The slowing down of body metabolism and a kind of default action to repair and survival mode accompanies food deprivation even for short periods. The authors comment at length on the efficacy advantages in the use of chemotherapy drugs in fighting cancer.

The writers also express the reason for IF as being an intention to fool the body into thinking that a state of potential famine has arrived and that it needs to go from a go-go mode to maintenance mode. The most compelling argument for it is the supposedly proven result of swift, sustainable weight loss while still allowing for consumption of a wide range of food types.

The 5:2 Plan

Mosley and Spencer also discuss their IF 5:2 plan which evolved from their experimentation with various versions of fasting and which they suggest guarantees success. The base principle is 5 days off of regular meals and 2 days on (such as Mondays and Thursdays) fasting for two non-consecutive days each week, allowing between 500 and 600 calories, each day split between breakfast and dinner. This approximates to ensuring two 12-hour periods without food within a 24-hour day. The plan allows for some modification within the basic framework; for example, breakfast later in the day (11:00 a.m.) and supper at 7:00 p.m. means fasting for 16 hours within a 24-hour period.

Food choices during fast days should be high protein with a low glycemic index. Boycotting carbs is not recommended. What looks like a mantra to retrain the brain is that on fast days "refrain, restrain, divert, and distract." It is noted that this 5:2 plan is devoid of rigid commandments in many respects.

The OMAD Pattern of Restricted Calorie Consumption

For the one meal a day (OMAD) IF, individuals choose different meals for their personal focus, such as dinner. This pattern of essentially fasting for 23 hours and eating one meal a day sure gives time for the stomach to rest. (Reportedly, in ancient times, samurais did not eat three meals a day; they had one huge meal at dinner.) Almost 200,000 Facebook followers dedicated to this fasting pattern share their experiences on the internet.

Data from one study indicates a 12% reduction in body fat mass compared to no change in a control group. An additional advantage was reduction in levels of the stress hormone cortisol, which can promote fat storage. It is suggested that important pointers for this fasting diet are ensuring consumption of enough food for daily sustenance and ensuring that intake takes place within a one-hour window Opinions differ on this advisability. [Hochwald 2022]

Drinks, such as sparkling water, broth in moderation, green tea, black coffee, and low-calorie beverages, are permitted outside the eating window within a 20-hour period. In this arrangement, high-calorie food consumption takes place within the remaining 4-hour window. Guidance is generally provided on the nature of meals including dairy and carbohydrates (Maxbauer, 2022).

Alternate Day Fasting

Alternative day fasting (ADF) caters for eating normally (regular, wholesome meals) one day and limited calories, such as 500 calories or less, the next day.

A Note on IF for Weight Control

If the information provided above relating to OMAD and various fasting ratios is of interest, further details relating to actual implementation must be carefully examined before commencing any programme. In the early trial of these options, an individual may experience a short temper and lack of concentration, but that these symptoms disappear within a month. Mental preparation is a must. Concerning the meal to skip, breakfast appears to be a better alternative; skipping dinner suggests less problems, apparently leading to less issues with sleep. It is also advisable to gradually increase fasting time day by day compared to fasting to aggressively at the start. Avoidance of overeating during non-fasting times and consulting with one's medical doctor are also advisable.

Supporters of fasting initiatives stress effective weight loss, reduction of risk relating to heart disease and stroke, and improved brain function. There seems, however, to be a lack of a clear consensus on what actually takes place during fasting and the unique benefits derived from the process. Some claim that it is equally beneficial to simply pursue daily caloric restriction. Travers [2022] makes the point that, in reality, IF is really a way of flipping the metabolism, as in the Keto diet, from using glucose to ketones. There is an indication that combining Keto and IF is a popular practice because of similarity in fat burning process.

Author Megan McMorris (2022) comments: "As long as you can do it correctly and healthfully, though, Fasting can be beneficial for weight loss, plus provide perks Like improvements in blood pressure and blood sugar levels."

Yang (2023), an experienced professional in various areas of medicine lists nine advantages of intermittent fasting:

1. Anti-aging
2. Weight loss
3. Igniting autophagy
4. Improving chronic disease
5. Increased exercise performance
6. Cancer prevention
7. Decreasing progression of Alzheimer's and Parkinson's diseases
8. Reduction in immune disease
9. Reduction of damage caused by concussion

Yang (2023) also provides three guiding commentaries on IF:

Keep Yourself Busy. Stay active and entertained during the period of fasting to keep distracted from stomach rumbles. However, avoid aggravating activities, such as grocery shopping. Reading, a family walk, and household chores are acceptable.

Don't Dwell on Hunger. Dismiss the misconception that one gets hungrier as time goes on. Over time, the body takes the calories it needs from body fat (from its own source) to feed itself. The hunger wave will pass.

Cut One Meal to Start. Do not enter all-in on to the fasting programme at the beginning. Start slowly, pushing back mealtimes gradually leading to dropping a meal. Do not add on missed calories later in the day. An example would be to start with 12 hours each of fasting and eating; then, consider shifting to a 16:8 schedule to move gradually to the longer fasting period.

SUMMARY

This chapter is in large measure a listing of information on selected diets, or more precisely diet-labelled plans or systems of aggressive management of food consumption intended to assist individuals struggling to control excess body weight, in particular. They are representative of, behavioural food intake patterns established in various communities over time. The core intention is to enable the pursuit of healthy and long-lasting lives. Variations in the more prominent and popular core systems are indicated.

The reader must take note, however, of the general conclusion that managing or improving one's diet is more significant and effective in the long run, compared to exercise by itself. It gives credence to the popular statement "you are what you eat."

An interesting article by S. F. Morell (2022) reviews research by a Dr. Weston Price, a dentist, on diet types as they relate to teeth and gum health in a wide range of different countries, given the understandable conflict which has emerged over time about a healthy diet. A major finding was that diets which sustained superb health may have differed in some particular features; however, their shared commonality was that none of them contained any processed or devitalized food of modern commerce. Animal foods and nutrient density items were also quite prominent in the compositions. The overall take away is very much not to deny that healthy diets may exist in any part of the world, including so-called primitive societies, but that the composition of the overall intake of what you eat (quality, balanced nutrients, and so forth), which supplies vital nutrients and ensures facilitation of adequate assimilation, is a major part of the answer.

Gottfried's (2021) commentary on the keto diet is clearly significant with respect to the range of diets being created and presented as the answer to the obesity tsunami: "Part of the problem with getting reliable and evidence-based information on the ketogenic diet is that we are witnessing an infodemic."

This applies to the undoubtedly difficult task in the search for trustworthy sources which can be used in the determination of ethical guiding principles for a wide range of individuals. It is clear that there is need for awareness that personal circumstances relating to congenital health conditions can affect metabolic reaction in different ways. Matters relating to kidney, pancreatic, and liver conditions can affect overall results. There is also the issue of differential unique hormonal needs of women and the effect on final outcomes as they relate to any particular individual.

Serious caution is needed in taking heed of the constant media bombardment suggesting a range of products guaranteed to do the impossible: lose weight without exercising! No dieting—safe and natural! There seems to be almost no limit to the language used to promote sales for "miracle" pills and drops, or herbs "from far off lands."

The increased shift to online shopping simply increases vulnerability of the average non-suspecting shopper. Some countries intervene at the official level having arrangements for staff of appropriate government bodies to execute internet surveillance for individuals or companies in violation of protective laws. Resources will inevitably be scarce, and it is best for consumers to be skeptical and to proceed with caution re trials with new "miracle" products and diets.

The weight loss industry has showered the anxious public with a massive array of products intended to help pop away excess fat. Many of them tout effective keto action, to "harness" the ketosis effect. A recent advert story on the internet relates to full team financing by the famous TV *Shark Tank* panel of investors. The packaged pill based upon scientific discovery by two sisters and marketed under the name "Keto Max Science" has received top rating out of a line-up of five similar fat loss supplements. It touts 70% increase in metabolism and zero negative side effects.

Similarly, among the fast and furious emerging discoveries is another "miracle" cure based on research by Harvard medical student Emily that claims to "fight against leptin resistance" (USA Today, 2023) and marketed under the name Thrive Keto ACV Gummies.

Readings of a more credible nature include information from Harvard Medical School which recently launched an online study programme which in essence indicates a need to remove the focus from dieting. The course, "Lose Weight and Keep It Off," has the tagline: "This easy-to-follow audiovisual roadmap can help you lose 10, 20, 30 pounds and more with no dieting, no starvation, no calorie-counting, and no deprivation." The course overview acknowledges the many stories of reported success with dieting initiatives but makes the point that ever so often, "life happens and, slowly but surely, the pounds creep back on and we're back where we started from...or even worse."0

The Harvard School of Medicine offers guidance incorporating results from evidence-based strategies that facilitate development of a tailored plan guaranteed to be effective. Overall, the resulting weight-loss plan embodies, inter alia, information relating to obesity causing bacteria, sugars, consumption of weight-busting fibre, good versus bad fats, brain confusion resulting from use of artificial sweeteners, mindful eating strategy, stress management, the problem of calorie-laden meals, and effective weight management habits.

It would appear , however, that we can not lose sight of the "gene" factor as we monitor results.

Researchers have made the [point that there is a "gene" effect which can pose challenges on an individual basis:

> Research has shown that our body's reaction to different diets
> and even television food advertising are influenced by genes.

If in search of general information, Walsh (2022) references four apps intended to facilitate fasting: Fastient, Zero, Body Fast, and Life Fasting Tracker—all available at varying prices.

It is quite clear: diet in and by itself holds no promise for effective weight management in the context of healthy living. Exercise is a part of the successful intervention on a sustained basis. Variables (diet and exercise) which can be controlled by the individual are much more significant in the control of obesity than all other factors including race, age, gender, and ethnicity. Further simplified: by Greger [2019], "Genes load the gun and lifestyle pulls the trigger."

In essence, adopt healthy habits and enjoy the benefits of good genes with positive lifestyle choices. The Harvard Report (2020) acknowledges that "aspects of diet play role in the prevention of disease and dysfunctions in almost every organ in the body" and that conservative consumption of a healthy diet reduces the risk of life-threatening diseases. In this regard, the HIIT labeled programs are more lifestyle changes than real diet applications; no foods are off limit.

At the end of the day, the overall summary conclusion lies with changes in lifestyle. The following statement by Rosemary Anderson (2022) gives expression to the underlying pointers which ultimately emerge for battling obesity:

> ...healthy living is a holistic endeavour. Knowing which foods are good for us is just one piece of the puzzle. The key to optimal health also includes exercise, socialization and... yes... eschewing a Western diet."

CHAPTER 7
GUT BACTERIA:
THE MICROBIOME

THE GUT IS the gastrointestinal tract which is the tube that starts at the mouth and ends at the other end! It must be a well-oiled machine, according to Cassie Irwin (2019). There is considerable referencing of gut bacteria, aka the microbiome or microbiota, in the literature on weight control. It has been referred to as the vast ecosystem of microbes existing largely in the large intestine. ,

References are made to gut bacteria in various sections of this book giving a clear indication of the broad relevance of the subject matter to good health, in general, and more specifically to the issue of obesity. This material is relevant, fascinating, and exhaustive. Readers, with perhaps limited or no real interest in science, will also find the material of interest. The reader will not be disappointed. Professionals consider the microbiome as being extremely important concerning digestion, nutrient absorption, and immunity surveillance. Available information strongly suggests a shift in focus by the large number of persons who fail to make progress on sustainable weight control after considerable expenditure of time and money on diets, the gym, and all kinds of exercise regimes.

A recent commentary (Littlemore, 2019) on *The Whole-Body Microbiome* illustrates the kind of holistic relevance to good health with respect to the microbiome: Research now links a healthy microbial balance to the performance of metabolic and immune functions which prevent disease development In essence, the human microbiome is regarded as "a frontier of modern medicine". [Denney, 2023]

> The microbial colonies in our bodies would seem to have some collaborative responsibility for every aspect of human health. The bacterial community—your personal microbiome—is one of the great predictors of a long and happy life.

Considerable information points to inflammation playing a very important role in many of the chronic diseases affecting human health; reportedly, in eight of the top ten leading causes of death (Greger, 2019). This widespread inflammation appears to be the reaction of our immune system to many of the unhealthy aspects of day-to-day life. Available data already suggest a microbial linkage with some 542 human diseases across more than 20 sites on the body. [Denney, April 13-19, 2023]

INFLAMMATION AND DISEASE IN THE HUMAN BODY: LEAKY GUT AND OTHER RELATED CONDITIONS

The non-elimination of waste products leads us to a condition of inflammation known as "leaky gut." The leakage relates to undigested food products crossing into the blood stream, eventually resulting in inflammation in different parts of the body, including the brain and the cardiovascular system. The condition is also described as "impaired intestinal permeability"; the mucosal lining of the digestive tract (in particular, the small intestine) loses its integrity and becomes permeable. Dr. Vincent Pedre says it's when you experience the silent epidemic, a deterioration of "border control."

There is also a toxic build-up of sludge, bacteria colonies, and parasites (bacterial overgrowth). This leads to overeating and faster colony growth. The result can include large, undigested protein food particles, pathogenic organisms, and various chemical circumstances passing through the leaking membrane as "foreign invaders" and entering the blood stream.

Both lectin and gluten are recognised "gut busters," leaking endotoxins storming across the entire body and leading to health problems in the joints, blood, heart tissue, and the death of brain cells. These gut busters rip apart the cells in the gut lining; the result is the underlying cause of most modern health issues.

By whatever name, the critical issue is the same: leakage between the usually tight cell junctions. These leaks inevitably lead to inflammation. Foul-smelling methane gas is a notable by-product.

An inflamed gut means that calcium and sodium are entering surrounding cells, causing them to attract and hold water. While attempting to flush toxins, the extra water lowers the function of the cells' energy centres (the mitochondria) and the body feels sluggish. This has the effect of tissue swelling and abdominal bloating. A major aspect of this condition is that the affected person looks much fatter than they really ought to look. It can give a bulging appearance to an individual of 10 to 25 pounds of excess fat.

It is not true fat! It is water-logged tissue. This condition is never corrected by ordinary weight loss diets.

The biggest culprit behind this inflammation related condition is processed foods. Reduced calorie and diet foods stoke the fire! They are full of chemicals and highly refined products. Diet sodas and frozen, low-calorie entrées are just about suicidal. Processed foods and animal products with high quantities of fat, trans-fats, and cholesterol are found to be pro-inflammatory compared to the anti-inflammatory qualities of whole plant foods such as fibre and phytonutrients.

Pro-inflammatory diets are especially associated with abdominal obesity. Fatty tissue actively secretes inflammatory chemicals into the blood stream and obesity leads to systemic inflammation. The top five sources of saturated fat in a Western diet include cheeses, desserts, chicken, pork, and burgers. All this is a clear indication of the need for definitive food choices in the pursuit of routine lifestyle: avoidance and limited, cautious consumption by individuals who are conscious of their personal obesity challenges.

It then becomes a priority matter that the individual makes every effort to reverse the inflammation by eliminating processed and packaged foods. The inflammation will calm down and the body will recalibrate. Recommendations include the use of grapes and green tea; also berries, dark leafy greens, and drinking lots of cold water.

One point of view is that leaky gut is a condition often missed by doctors; the result being that large numbers of people have no idea of the nature of the problem (*First for Women*, 2016).

It is clearly a kind of hot spot with respect to unsuccessful or difficult weight management issues. Don Colbert (2021), celebrated nutritionist and medical practitioner, refers to leaky gut as a "simple problem with devastating effects, one that can make it impossible to lose weight." His treatment programme for tackling what he calls "stubborn pounds of belly fat" focuses on repairing the gut lining and reducing the passing through of the "sneaky evil endotoxins." This also brings relief to conditions of bloating and gas accumulation.

Leaky gut syndrome is almost always associated with autoimmune disease, a condition in which the immune system accidentally attacks one's body instead of protecting it. A damaged gut is a common source of chronic inflammation since up to 80% of the immune system is located in the gut.

Funk (2020) illustrates the potential significance of this particular gut condition:

> Almost every disease—from depression tyuo anxiety, obesity, autoimmune disease, or heart disease—and the related symptoms that go with so many ailments—are associated with the health of your gut… I originally thought that leaky gut was an isolated condition affecting a few unfortunate individuals, now I am convinced that leaky gut underlies all our disease just as Hippocrates posited.

A leaky gut may well be associated with "leaky brain" also, implying some relationship with Alzheimer's and Parkinson's.

HEALING THE GUT

Given the potential danger of a leaky gut condition, it is important to heal the situation. Colbert (2021) focuses on a "healthy gut zone"; its significance in what I choose to call "human health globality" is indicated by the subtitle: *Heal Your Digestive System to Restore Your Body and Renew Your Mind.*

He emphasises the importance of avoiding foods which are lectin rich, such as GMO foods and foods full of gluten.

There is a long list of food products to be avoided or minimized in the healing of leaky gut. It appears advisable to focus on removing the things that cause the inflammation to break the dangerous cycle since the body tends to crave the very foods that bring on the condition. They either damage the gut, contribute to inflammation, or boost the presence of bad bacteria in the gut.

Recommendations from different sources amount to a formidable list of don'ts or preferred avoidance, including:

1. Avoid damaging sources, including processed, fast foods, sugar and caffeine, all soy products, and GMO foods.
2. Avoid or minimize the use of grains (barley, rye, wheat, oats, rice, even quinoa). All are high in lectin. Millet and sorghums do not contain gluten. It is interesting to note that white basmati rice is lower in lectins than other rice varieties. The general principle is to eliminate gluten, a highly inflammatory protein.
   a. It is further advised to soak legumes for 24 hours, discarding the water, and cook in a pressure cooker to reduce of the lectin effect.
3. Colbert (2017) advises that persons with autoimmune disease should avoid gluten forever and be concerned with the how dairy products containing milk protein are consumed. Appropriate dietary advice is indicated. The casein in dairy provokes autoimmunity. Some sources suggest avoiding dairy products (cheese, cream, milk, butter, yogurt, and so forth) and also avoiding the effect of growth hormones used by farmers.
4. Eliminate or reduce saturated fats (butter, cheese, cream, and coconut oil).
5. Eggs, a common allergen, can create inflammation.
6. Avoid nuts; seeds; seed fruits; such as squash, zucchini, cucumbers, and pumpkin; beans, peas, and especially lentils.

7. Avoid nightshade plants which contain small quantities of alkaloids: tomatoes, eggplants, potatoes, and peppers; however, discarding seed and skins removes the lectins. The same holds for seed fruits.
8. High-lectin foods.
9. Processed foods (most foods in a box) and excessive starches and carbs (potatoes, rice, corn). One recommendation is to limit starches to the size of a tennis ball per meal.
10. Minimise meat intake including chicken, beef, pork, and also processed meats.

Quite clearly, dietary choice when dealing with the healing of leaky gut presents a formidable, daily challenge. Keep in mind that the overall goal in seeking to heal the gut includes regaining a proper good versus bad bacterial balance, heal the holes in the gut wall, and to quench inflammation.

DIVERSITY (GOOD VERSUS BAD) OF BACTERIA

There is considerable information on bacteria types which one will find to be of interest. More than 2,000 species of bacteria have been identified in the human microbiome. Reportedly, there is a kind of individuality, and yet a range, in the bacterial assembly within the gut flora. There are apparently two types of human gut flora: those who grow mostly Bacteroides species and those who grow mostly Prevotella.

Panoff (2020) comments on the range of environmental circumstances which determine the make-up of your gut bacteria:

> a community of bacteria that is unique to you from before birth… your microbiome is altered throughout your life by your lifestyle and personal habits… the places you spend time, your environmental exposures, your diet, how much you exercise, the medications you take, other health conditions, and even mental stress can influence what your microbiome looks like. As such, your gut bacteria typically looks very different from that of the people around you, especially if you live very different lifestyles.

We can all benefit from a little information on the significance of bacteria in the functional operation of the human body. Greger[2019] is an excellent source for some simplified and meaningful information. He makes the point that our "obesogenic" (obesity-generating) environment is not to be ignored and that individuals vary in their susceptibility to the condition. All indications are that genetic variation plays only a small part with respect to body size when this condition is expressed. It appears that another source of genetic material may provide the answer It may well be closely associated with the DNA contained in all the variety of different microbes that inhabit our bodies, most of which live inside our gut.

Any attempt to answer what the benefits are to the body housing these "tenant" organisms in the microbiome is provided by the following statements:

> Rent is paid in the form of boosting our immune systems, balancing our hormones, improving digestion, and making vitamins for us… our gut flora don't just constitute any organ but perhaps the main organ involved in the cause of obesity. [Greger 2019]

The majority of bacteria in the gut originate from the vaginal flora acquired from the mother at birth. Interestingly, children born by caesarean section commence life with a bacterial population more resembling that of the operating room, a possible explanation of why children born via this procedure "have a 33 percent greater risk of childhood obesity." Another author references a 25% higher risk of obesity, the same for asthma and diabetes. This indicates that the first and best birthday present for the newborn is received in the form of "the vaginal and fecal microbes they ingest and collect moving down the birthing canal" (Littlemore, 2019/ Greger 2019].

Recent research from Finland indicates significant effect on "the composition of infant gut microbes" as a result of chronic prenatal psychological distress of mothers. Concerns relate to infant growth and development as well as a possible association with disease risk later in life.

One possible medical procedure under consideration to correct this disadvantage is "vaginal seeding" involving the transfer of material from vaginal fluids to newborn caesarean babies to provide a more natural flora. Breast-fed babies, benefiting from special compounds in breast milk which nourish their microbiome, are less likely to display obese childhood patterns. In the same context, there are already references to a possible last-resort treatment of highly resistant bad gut bacteria by resorting to a "slurry up" of selected healthy donor feces for injection or enema application in a re-population process (Littlemore, 2019).

There are references to good and bad bacteria in quite a few publications where the matter of the microbiome is discussed. This differentiation is highlighted to a larger extent where the discussion on weight control shifts to pre- and pro-biotics. Further discussion on these preparations follows later.

There are no lack of indications of the far-reaching significance of gut bacteria. Research findings suggest some impact on the performance of marathon runners in that certain types of bacteria are more prevalent in the context of good performance (Hicklin, 2019).

It is critical to ensure plenty of good bacteria outbalancing the bad bacteria. A predominance of bad bacteria is known as dysbiosis and has been found to contribute to depression and Alzheimer's disease via oxidative stress. This refers to cell and tissue damage resulting from an imbalance in harmful free radicals and protective antioxidants.

PERSONAL POO AND HUMAN HEALTH

Personal poo is not generally discussed in most cultures, at least not in polite company. Hopefully, after reading this book, you will regard what exits your body (assuming your elimination is functioning properly and "the stuff" is not being deposited as fat on your waist, buttocks, and so forth) as being just as important as what you take in. Gerasimo (2017) suggests a basic fact never to be forgotten:

> Your poo offers a view into your state of well being. Basically, if the stuff coming out of you isn't in optimal form, it suggests that some things inside of you aren't going as well as they

could, either… most people don't have a lot of information to draw on regarding what is and is not considered good in the world of poo.

That exit material from the human body is the primary pathway through which the body flushes waste and can reveal the health of the intestinal system in general, and more specifically provides information on our digestion, nutrient assimilation, food sensitivities, levels of body inflammation, the presence or absence of important pathogens, cancers, autoimmune disorders, and more. In essence, our traditional hurried glance into the toilet bowl can be more informative than you would have thought before reading this book.

I have already warned you that in an obese condition, negative influences pile up; there is a backing up and fermentation, and the situation produces waste products of its own referred to as "endogenous waste." Once again, the focal concern becomes the gut lining. The "stuff" can leak through the lining and, inter alia, lead to interference with hormonal, neurologic, and immune functions. Stagnant stool is a negative in weight management. The result is irritation, inflammation and permeability issues of the intestinal lining with all the range of possible health conditions referred to elsewhere in this review.

In advancing medicine, poo matters. New medical initiatives have commenced its usage as a form of medication. Healthy stool samples are introduced into the colon associated with a defective intestine by a procedure known as fecal transplant to repopulate with good bacteria. The procedure may involve use of an enema or use of a pill to be swallowed.

In the struggle against obesity, the obese individual must understand fully that pooping does not help weight loss. Any noticeable loss in weight after a large BM is insignificant. It is mostly water loss and temporary. Relevant variables in the frequency of BM are water, fibre intake, body size, and diet.

There are two different types of fibre: soluble (oat bran, nuts, beans) and insoluble (wheat bran, vegetables, whole grain). The former slows digestion while the latter aids the bulking of stool and facilitates quick passage. Intake of soluble fibre lowers the risk of visceral belly fat.

Obesity is associated with a higher risk of abnormal bowel movements; there seems to be a 60% more likely risk of chronic diarrhoea[- (Ballou et. al, 2019).

Assessment of stool quality involves determination of one's stool microbiological profile. Some countries do use fecal transplants to treat gut-related sicknesses and disease. Research results in Copenhagen, Sweden, suggest that fecal intestinal transplants may be effective against obesity— and type 2 diabetes.

PREBIOTICS AND PROBIOTICS

Prebiotics and probiotics feature quite significantly in the attempt to manage issues relating to the human gut flora which make up the microbiome. With tons of information and numerous offers about the best products on which to spend your money, I attempt to provide some fundamental information.

Healing the gut requires four core dietary inclusions: prebiotics, probiotics, fibre, and polyphenols. The latter are plant-derived substances with a stress-reducing capability. They boost the immune system and facilitate proper brain function, and are also effective in guarding against diabetes and gastrointestinal disorders. Pomegranate juice is highlighted as a rich source. Other sources include berries, chestnuts, dark chocolate, coffee, cocoa powder, green tea, olive oil, and olives. Adding polyphenols to the diet assists in weight loss by inhibiting fat cell development.

Probiotics are simply live organisms (bacteria and yeasts) which are considered important in the health of the digestive system. They promote a healthy digestive tract which is critical to a functioning healthy immune system.

Numerous sources exist on probiotics, so it may be of help to have some knowledge now before facing with a multitude of choices on store shelves. Reportedly, probiotics represent a 35-billion-dollar industry. Sources of probiotics include:
- Fermented foods (some pickles, sauerkraut, kimchi, tempeh)
- Juices with good bacteria strains added

- Some cheeses, such as cottage cheese, Gouda, cheddar, moz-
  zarella; all of which typically maintain good bacteria during the
  ageing process
- Fermented and unfermented milk, buttermilk, kefir (a yogurt-
  like drink)
- Kombucha (a fermented tea or drink with live organisms)

Yogurt has been referred to as the best-known probiotic food, and especially plain yogurt. Live active cultures can be a powerful source of probiotics in dealing with type 2 diabetes. On reaching the gut, the probiotics
within assist in regulating blood glucose levels. Some writers recommend
the intake of probiotic foods at least once a day.

Panoff (2021) remarks that it can be overwhelming in making choices
regarding which probiotic to try. It is clearly advantageous to have some
understanding of how these products support good health. The composition of a person's digestive bacteria is subject to daily alteration. It is, therefore, extremely important to be continuously facilitating the presence of
good bacteria colonies in top condition within your gut microbiome.

The regular addition of probiotics to your diet facilitates the maintenance of a healthy ratio of good bacteria. This initiative supposedly impacts
one's overall health, supporting the immune system together with digestive
and mental health. Impacting the digestive system conveys significance in
the struggle against obesity. Quite often, individuals turn to probiotics for
relief with conditions relating to gas and abdominal bloating, diarrhoea,
and mild stomach upset.

The use of antibiotics can impact negatively both good and bad gut
bacteria, killing them off and possibly resulting in diarrhoea when used
for bacterial infections. Probiotics provide a buffer in these situations by
populating the gut with good bacteria. Most probiotics contain at least two
species of bacteria, primarily Lactobacillus and Bifidobacterium. They are
targeted for research with respect to their impact on weight control. It is
indicated that specific strains affect the human body with different results.

The potential for new advances in probiotic production and recent
references to vaginal seeding of the human microbiome have already
been discussed within this chapter. Future research may identify and

target problematic and beneficial microbes, producing tailored probiotics. Indeed, a whole new range of probiotics could gain interest, given the potential for microbiome alteration in the absence of our ability to alter our genetics.

Probiotics and Mental Health

While mental health is not the focus of this book, given the critical importance of the microbiome to one's general well-being, I consider it useful to draw attention, briefly, to an interesting connection between probiotics and mental health. Brix (2020) writes about the "gut-brain axis," the point being the existence of an intricate connection between these two organs; for example, reference to a gut-wrenching reaction or mouth salivation when one thinks of eating something special. In all these reactions, the gut microbiome plays a critical role; communication takes place between the enteric nervous system in the gut and the central nervous system in the brain. She writes:

> Many recent studies reveal that this bacterial community is connected to a person's mental health, and there is a link between gut health and the development of mental disorders such as depression and anxiety.

Research data points to more than average numbers of individuals with irritable bowel syndrome (IBS) developing depression and anxiety. Brix's article (2020) is somewhat unique in the way she brings to the fore the significance of soluble fibre working in combination with both prebiotics and probiotics. Meals high in soluble fibre and supplemented with the other two facilitate the presence of good bacteria and support the axis of digestive and mental/emotional health. In addition, the presence of soluble "prebiotic fibre" slows digestion, increases satiety and helps to regulate blood sugar.

Prebiotics assist in modulating emotional stresses and stress responses. It would appear impossible to overemphasise the importance of gut bacteria in achieving and maintaining superb human health... Brix,2020 emphasizes the range of importance of a strong and healthy gastrointestinal tract

How to Take Probiotics

The science on the use and effectiveness of probiotics would appear to be unsettled in some respects. Results appear to be affected by strain, composition, dosing, and intention. Reportedly, probiotics may work differently for men and women; it is even suggested that they may offer more success in the support for long-term weight loss for females.

Newcomers to the use of probiotics may experience side effects of bloating, loose stool, or gas; these conditions are likely to be short term (a few days). The gradual increase of dosages is suggested. Both frequency and length of time for taking probiotics are for consideration. On both issues, consultation with a competent health provider is recommended for guidance on maintaining an overall healthy gut microbiome.

Probiotic supplements are available in different forms, usually as a capsule or powder. With regard to what qualifies as the most effective antibiotic, Panoff (2020) states that:

> it can depend on a number of factors, such as the Strain of bacteria in the product, how many bacteria It contains, how the probiotic is stored, whether the Product contains prebiotics, and what condition You're looking to target.

The inclusion of both pre- and probiotics in the formulation is an advantage. My personal experience in nutrition shops is that one seldom finds an attendant who can give professional guidance on matters of this nature; numerous sources have already been indicated above.

Caution is suggested when taking probiotics.; usage is not recommended together with antibiotics, the latter being dispensed to kill bacteria. A 2- to 3-hour spacing is recommended to minimise negative reactions including the probiotics being rendered useless (Colbert, 2019). Some writers recommend probiotic foods at least once a day.

Safety of Probiotics

Some research studies have raised concerns about the safety of probiotics, and in some cases it has been concluded that they cannot be considered harmless. In some cases, there is an indication of assisting weight gain.

Overall, modest benefits are indicated. The individual must be cautious in making choices among the numerous combinations and dosages of probiotic material on the market

PREBIOTICS

Prebiotics have been referred to as a "food, fuel or fertilizer for probiotics and gut bacteria" (Baxter, 2021). They are dietary fibrous compounds required by probiotics to thrive adequately in the gut. They feed the good bacteria and facilitate good health by supporting metabolism and digestion, two critical body functions in weight control, in general, more so in the obesity challenge. Together, they are immunity boosters.

In the chapter on diets, within the context of sweeteners, you were introduced to yacon syrup, a newly touted replacement for already known natural and artificial sweeteners. Its indigestible fibre and low-sugar content make it a prize inclusion among prebiotics which are crucial for the establishment of good gut bacteria. Effective prebiotic supplements are characterized by the content of fibre, resistant starch, and the presence of sugars in the form of fructans, generally undigestible and not contributing to fat accumulation but very welcome by the good and friendly gut flora.

Prebiotics pass through the GI tract undigested and make their way to the gut where they catch up with the probiotics. Together, they form a formidable team for fighting off bad bacteria and facilitating the cultivation of good bacteria.

Prebiotics can be found naturally in a variety of foods. Indicated sources include garlic, leeks, onions, asparagus, barley, bananas, Jerusalem artichokes, oats, cocoa, apples, flax seed, beans, jicama, seaweed, chicory root, honey, maple syrup, and even red wine is now included (Karst, 2023).

Sources of these products available for purchase abound under different brand names in pharmacies, nutrition shops, via the internet, and so forth. They can be purchased separately packaged or in combination.

Advertisements may offer:

"Unique 9 strain formula… 55 billion live probiotic cultures" (Calton and Jayson, 2017)

"Organic Indian yogurt smoothie… grass fed… 60 billion live probiotics"

"Travel biotic 10 billion" (Calton and Jayson, 2017)

"True potency probiotic… one clinically proven strain… 30 billion"

PLANT-BASED FOODS AND GUT HEALTH

One important dietary to which individuals appear to be turning increasingly: weight management achieved through emphasis on plant-based diets. Chapter 8 has a focus on this very important subject matter.

SUMMARY

The gut bacteria are increasingly a research focus for general health and the management of obesity. Much of the work is still in its infancy. There is, however, already considerable evidence that the nature and condition of your microbiome are linked with issues of obesity and a range of other health issues, possibly including mental illness. This chapter provides considerable insight into possible stubborn fat loss and the condition known as leaky gut, a condition which may not be diagnosed but if present, demands special attention.

The importance of probiotics and prebiotics is introduced and important considerations in using them are indicated.

CHAPTER 8
PLANT-BASED WHOLE FOODS AND CALORIE DENSITY: ELEMENTS OF CONTROL FOR EFFECTIVE DIETARY PATTERNS

CALORIES: ITS PROMINENCE IN THE MANAGEMENT OF OBESITY

THE GENERAL CONCLUSION, in the context of human nutrition, is that there is an explosion in obesity, perhaps more so in Western countries, and especially in North America; it is a kind of global epidemic. The simple explanation is that there is a definite shift in dietary patterns towards consuming more calories accompanied by a reduction in physical activity.

Leaving out the current distortion in production and transportation issues arising from the global COVID-19 crisis, the situation in North America is that of an explosion over the past 3 to 4 decades in the per-capita production of calories. Generally, this means lots more of available food. This expanded production, in part, accounts for heavier children and adults and expanded waistlines. Other related causes include increased portion sizes, especially in restaurants, adult individuals spending more time as "couch potatoes" while looking at television or playing video games, as well as a paucity of exercise opportunities in the curriculum of schools. It all adds up to increased calorie intake in dietary patterns with the excess calories being deposited as body fat.

Another important part of the explanation is that while obese individuals do not necessarily eat large amounts of food, the new dietary habits in food choices mean more calories per mouthful. This becomes a reality of overeating because the selected foods are abnormally and unnaturally loaded or dense in calories.

Calorie density refers to the number of calories represented by a given weight or volume of food. In essence, some foods have more calories per unit of space (per pound, per mouthful, and so forth) compared to other food items.

What Is a Calorie?

The word "calorie" represents a unit of measurement, a significant point of reference as we discuss food intake, both quantity and quality. The basic scientific explanation is that it is the amount of heat needed to raise the temperature of one gram of water by one degree Celsius.

The foods we consume provide essential energy so that our bodies can function. We eat in the first instance to sustain life. Even at this point, we must understand that if we take in too many calories, there is a risk of gaining weight. If the excess is not expended in physical activity, it will end up being dumped on our hips, waistlines, belly fat, and so forth.

Used with reference to food consumption, the relationship is tied to large calories. A kilocal equals kcal; one kilocalorie being equivalent to 1,000 small calories. We have already learnt that all calories are not the same.

CALORIC CONSUMPTION: DIVERSITY IN VOLUME AND DENSITY—ADEQUATE OR EXCESSIVE?

The insulin-blood sugar management of obesity has been discussed at length and reviewed in earlier chapters. The relevance is anchored in the chemistry of human metabolism, including the activity of gut bacteria. Analysis of the obesity problem, however, from the point of view of calories consumed is also very relevant as we pursue a wholistic explanation for the average individual in search of what is appropriate daily behaviour for obesity management.

Pritikin's publication on the calorie density solution hammers home the case of calorie consciousness in the management of food intake and weight management. Selected quotes from the author conveys the core reasoning for his emphasis on the calorie-based approach:

> you want to know the average calorie density of your entire meal… ask ourselves an important question… how can I fill up my stomach, satisfy my hunger, and still lose weight… Meals composed of low calorie dense foods fill your stomach on significantly fewer calories than meals composed of high calorie dense foods.

THE EASE OF CONSUMING DIETARY EXCESS CALORIES: USING CALORIE DENSITY AS A GUIDE

Different food items provide different levels of energy. The three major macronutrients in our food chain are not equal in terms of calorie supply. Carbohydrates and proteins provide less than half the amount of calories per gram compared to fat. They differ in calorie density.

Complete frustration with a lack of success is the story reported quite frequently by individuals who embark on all kinds of initiatives to lose weight and reduce obesity. There is an adequate explanation in almost all such cases. What is quite obvious, however, is that most individuals seem to lack understanding of the full story of weight control with particular reference to what goes into their mouths, especially as it relates to their prevailing lifestyles.

Consuming about 150 calories can be accomplished by eating one candy bar or 30 cups of lettuce—a ton of difference as a human being, but the same number of calories. Understand, even at this stage, that the thinking must relate to whether the food item consumed supplies vitamins, fibre, or minerals, or if it is void of nutrients, full of "empty" of calories.

The above information is necessary in ensuring a thorough understanding of what follows in this chapter. More importantly, if obesity management is your goal, you should understand the varying levels of stupidity at which one can consciously choose to intake in frequency and quantity certain kinds of foods for daily dietary sustenance.

Let's illustrate the situation with a few examples:

1. One tablespoon of drizzled oil on a salad adds 120 calories, compared to 2 to 3 cups of berries (equal in calories) which will fill the average stomach.
2. A handful of jelly beans carries about six times the amount of calories in 4 cups of cherry tomatoes.
3. Consider the ever-popular French fries: a small serving carries the same number of calories as a small baked potato. A large serving has the calorie equivalent to about four baked potatoes.
4. The "willpower booby trap" is demonstrated if you go to the gym, sweat for 1 hour, and have lunch that fries with a sandwich; a classic case of flawed arithmetic: burn 300 calories and gobble up 500!
5. About 2 pints of strawberry ice cream is roughly 2,000 calories, the equivalent of about 40 cups of berries which belong to the low-calorie-density group.

Looking at comparative quantities of selected food items on a volume basis, see the quantity of broccoli one would have to consume to match the same number of calories of certain, the approximate figures can be surprising:

chick peas x8	oatmeal x5
cashew nuts x20	watermelon balls x1+
butter x50	sweet potato cubes x5
cookies x32	chicken x16
9 eggs x5	cheese x34

This explains the popularity of broccoli for weight management; these food items are many times more calorie dense compared to consuming broccoli. Fill up with broccoli, feel full, and keep the consumption of calories low for weight management.

Two other popular low-calorie-density food items used for this purpose are zucchini and cucumbers. The high water content of kale and apple slices also make them desirable for the same purposes. The simple lesson here is make cucumber, kale, and zucchini your close friends. Do not forget the value of inclusion of lettuce and the combination of spring mix leafy greens usually available in the supermarkets.

Consuming large quantities of selected foods allows the obese person to fill up, eat right, and still lose weight. If you consume 2–3 pounds of food based on eggs, meat, bread, and cheese, comparative calorie consumption on a healthy diet means approximately 12–13 pounds of vegetables or 4–5 pounds of starchy vegetables. Losing weight means that the obese person must deliberately make healthy choices.

PLANT-BASED DIETS AND GUT BACTERIAL COMPOSITION

Firstly, a brief look back once again at the microbiome (gut bacteria) and the significance of fibre- eating bacteria. We already know that the food choices we make affect the growth of trillions of bacteria in our microbiome; it determines which bacteria will persist and what they manufacture. Some bacteria types seem to be more evident than others when a comparison is made between obese and non-obese individuals. Studies have shown that those bacteria which appear to be protective against obesity eat fibre. There is a particular hormone, fasting-induced adipose factor, which comes into play when we fast; the body stops storing fat and initiates a burning off (Greger,2019). Some bacteria repress this hormone thereby facilitating fat storage, while the fibre-eating bacteria, makers of short-chain fatty acids, boost production of this particular hormone.

Consumption of fibre-rich foods has a double advantage. This promotes the presence of fibre-eating bacteria which produce a supply of short-chain fatty acids. In turn, these acids have a positive effect on the hormone mentioned above. Research points to the fact that consumption of plant-based foods results in colon flora with three times the capacity to produce these beneficial short-chain fatty acids.

Bacteria differ in relation to what is referred as the energy harvest. The obesity-related bacteria have a higher capability to break down human waste, harvest the calories, and send them back for reabsorption into the blood stream, reducing the effort to get rid of extra calories. Other bacteria have a reduced harvesting capacity and can better extract calories from our gut contents.

These findings apparently help to explain the advantage in weight control of persons who eat more of a plant-based diet. Analysis of feces of vegetarians tell the story.

Further review of the gut bacteria story becomes even more fascinating. It would appear that in human beings there are two basic gut bacteria types which are cultivated. This means two types of ecosystems; one grows a lot of Bacteroides, associated largely with the consumption of animal foods (fat, cholesterol, animal protein). The other grows a lot of the Prevotella bacteria species associated mostly with plant foods. The Prevotella are the fibre eaters; they produce short-chain fatty acids associated with more manageable weight control. The following statement summarises the core point to be made: "Native Africans who eat largely plant-based diets tend to have a Prevotella enterotype, while African Americans eating a typical Western diet tend to be in the Bacterioides camp." There can be considerable difference in calorie density between the typical African diet and a diet based upon Western-style fast food.

A very interesting observation from research data for persons considering switching to a plant-based diet is the rate at which the predominant type of bacteria switches with a change in diet. The apparently absolutely fastest rate for the bacterial switch following a change in diet is "as soon as the food hits our colons"—within 24 hours.

MANAGING FOOD-INTAKE CHOICES: GLUTEN AND GLYCEMIC INDEX

Before proceeding further with the broad discussion on plant-based foods, information is being provided on three selected topics, all of which help the reader to understand different outcomes in bodily appearance and health, depending on the extent to which food intake is guided by this additional knowledge. The information facilitates understanding the explanation behind dietary choices focussed on whole-plant foods. The topical areas include the fibre content of foods and also, the presence of gluten and the importance of glycemic measurements (glycemic index; glycemic load) of different food types. The ultimate objective, of course, is to provide important information aimed at facilitating modified behaviour, as may be advantageous for the individual seeking guidance in the management of obesity.

Glycemic Index and Plant-Based Foods

Treating obesity and related dietary-composition issues effectively requires an understanding of how and why different foods affect blood sugar levels and, therefore, their propensity to facilitate fat deposition.

The brain and the body, in general, prefer glucose (blood sugar) to function; however, too much too fast is both dangerous and unhealthy. Different carbohydrates affect blood sugar differently, and these effects can be quantified by measurement. The rating terms applicable here are glycemic index (GI) and glycemic load (GL). Both measurements are similar in purpose but one tells a little more than the other and, therefore, provides more of the full story in relation to the effect on your health. Either one will indicate how quickly food is broken down during digestion and, therefore, provide an indication of how quickly the food item causes an increase in blood glucose levels. As will be seen, this information guides choice in the inclusion or avoidance of different foods.

GI ratings range from 1–100. The rating is based on how much of a particular food has to be eaten to yield 50 grams of carbohydrate and how those 50 grams will cause your blood sugar level to rise. Pure glucose has a rating of 100. The higher the number on the GI scale, the more rapidly the carbohydrate of that food is converted to sugar and released. A low GI-scale measurement means a slow and steady release of glucose. A high GI indicates rapid release. Low GI foods contain more fibre and fat, foster weight loss, and are definitely more desirable for weight management.

Understanding GL is just as important as the GI rating when trying to understand the full story to the effect on blood sugar. GL also gives a rating of the amount of carbohydrate in a serving of food.

A summary rating for GI versus GL, together with some illustrative examples, is provided hereunder.

	GI	vs	GL
A	HIGH (more than 70) M--- cold breakfast cereals, breads, potatoes, rice snack chips Easy of ------ digestion, convert to blood glucose quickly Significant rise from blood glucose about 40–45 minutes after eating; capture substantive fluctuations		(more than 20) Dates------, white rice, corn flakes, baby potatoes, French fries, refined breakfast cereal, sugar-sweetened beverages (---) Couscous (1 cup) White basmati rice (1 cup cooked) White flour pasta (½ cup cooked)
B	MODERATE (45–70) A variety of foods including ice cream, orange juice, cakes, carbs, pizza		(11-19) Oatmeal, 1 cup cooked, spaghetti, sweet potatoes, bulgar, rice cakes, whole grain breads (1 slice); Whole grain pasta (¼ cup cooked)
C	LOW (below 11) Yogurt, pasta, milk, cooked dry beans, nuts, vegetables, ---- fruits, table sugar (sucrose), fruit sugar (fructose), whole oats, (slow digestion, prompting a slower riser in blood sugar)		(Less than 10) Kidney beans, fruit, whole grain, lentils, skim milk, cashews, peanuts, carrots, apples, oranges, bran cereals.

The question arises as to how this detailed information provides guidance on food-intake decisions in the effort to manage obesity.

The role of the pancreas and its supply of insulin as blood sugar rises has been clarified earlier, and we learnt that good health requires the blood sugar level to be controlled and remain fairly consistent. Also, that excess sugar is stored as fat. This means that as far as possible, blood sugar spikes are to be avoided in the management of obesity.

Simply speaking, focus your dietary intake on foods with lower GI ratings, say between 0 and 55 on the GI scale. Medium-rated foods can also be selected in second place. Keep in mind that a high GI rating means foods heavy in starch and that minimal consumption is advised. Rapid rises in blood sugar mean more fat is stored on the body. A GI below 45 means that they are slower in raising blood sugar.

When GL comes into the picture in the management of obesity, preferential food choices include those with a low GL rating of between 11 and 19 given that blood sugar spikes will not be sustained for long periods. GL loads that are higher mean a signal for very limited consumption in the diet of an obese person. Take note that low readings in both scales tend to go together.

The Harvard University Medical School website explains the relationship between the two rankings:

> The glycemic index tells just part of the story. What it doesn't tell you is how high your blood sugar could go when you actually eat the food. To understand a food's complete effect on blood sugar, you need to know both how quickly it makes glucose enter the blood stream and how much glucose per serving it can deliver... the Glycemic Load does both—which gives a more accurate picture of a food's real-life impact on your blood sugar.

Take a look at the reasoning behind the use of these two rating scales. The GI reading is based on the effect of a 50-gram serving of the particular food type. This means that it provides a more accurate picture of a particular food's real-life impact on blood sugar spikes.

For example, watermelon has a high glycemic index of 80 but this relates to a very small serving of carbohydrates. Given that 1 cup (154 grams) of watermelon yields only 11.6 grams of carbohydrates, it will require more than 4 cups (approx. 46 grams) of watermelon to yield the 50 grams of carbohydrate, the basic measuring standard of the GI system. It is considered unrealistic to anticipate a consumption of 50 grams of watermelon at a single serving. Its glycemic load ranking is only 5 and as a result the blood sugar rise will not be sustained for a long period.

We care about how quickly carbohydrates are digested because there is an effect on our appetites (metabolic rates) and, therefore, the amount of fat we burn. We already know that carbohydrates are a major concern in weight management; in addition, we need to be aware of the form in which they enter our mouths. Fruit, pasta, or candy different impacts have on our health.

Never lose sight of the end product of my SOB cousins: starch and sugar!

Higher blood sugar levels go with a higher frequency of sugar and insulin spikes. Lower glycemic foods provide longer periods of feeling full and minimize food appetite and are also associated with burning more fat.

A high glycemic diet is associated with higher levels of fat storage, even with the same number of calories. Consumption of 50% more calories than required on a high-glycemic diet can lead to a quarter-pound addition of pure fat to your body each day. The same number of extra calories on a low-glycemic diet can result in a 40% less addition of fat, about a pound of fat per week.

The significant lesson here is that depending on one's level of obesity, the individual has to understand the need for a critical level of consciousness which becomes necessary every time they place food in the mouth that will lead to a rise or spike in blood sugar. A red light must go on for food items such as ice cream, white flour, baked goods, cookies, all forms of pure sugar at breakfast, use of condensed milk in the morning coffee or afternoon tea, and consumption of aerated drinks and candy.

The easiest way to lean towards low-index foods is to focus on foods that are grown, not made. We then begin to understand why the increasing emphasis on whole-grain plant foods in the battle against obesity.

Hopefully, we are also now in a better position to understand the section that follows later in the chapter as it relates to the significance of gluten and fibre in the composition of foods consumed by an already obese person.

GLUTEN

There is increasing awareness of gluten in issues of excess fat and obesity. Currently, there is reference to the gluten craze with about 25% of the

U.S. population trying to avoid its consumption since it is regarded as a "problematic food compound" (Greger, 2019). Reportedly, there are some 10,000 products on the market now labelled as gluten-free.

Gluten is a general name for the family of proteins found in most grain products such as rye, barley, farina, semolina, triticale, and especially wheat products. It is referred to as a kind of "glue" which provides "squishiness or elasticity" to the particular food products and is common in bread, pasta, pizza, and cereal. Corn, rice, and the increasingly popular quinoa also contain gluten, but reportedly of a different type.

Some individuals are cautious with gluten since it can present some difficulty for use as a source of protein in the human body; it is then largely unusable and can cause difficulty through misdiagnosis by the body's immune system, leading to inflammation. Our gastrointestinal system can be regarded as being designed to work like a "closed system" with check points which facilitate the crossover of nutrients into the normal systemic location.

Gluten is reported to have a particular protein, gliadin, which can lead to openings or junction "leaks"—that is, when cells open too much, allowing large protein pieces to enter the blood stream with a resulting inflammatory immune action. The damaged intestine is compromised and experiences lower absorption of fat, fat-soluble vitamins, and micronutrients from food, all of which end up in stool without any absorption. The latter condition is known as "leaky gut", a condition already discussed at length early in the previous chapter.

Gluten can also impact weight loss, lower bone mineral density, cause iron and vitamin D deficiency, and can even cause neurological disorders.

Some individuals develop gluten intolerance, also called celiac disease, an autoimmune disease in which gluten triggers immune system activity. When it comes into contact with the inner lining of the small intestine, it causes inflammation and damage to the absorptive surface. This damage prevents absorption of nutrients. Reportedly, one in 133 Americans, mostly women, are sensitive to gluten and are advised to cut it out of their diet. Removal from the diet means a loss of good fibre; however, this can be made up by an increased intake of leafy vegetables and legumes.

Weight loss is one of the claimed benefits of a gluten-free diet. Sweet potato, a starchy vegetable, together with brown and wild rice, sorghum, and legumes are also gluten-free. For dietary purposes, one should be aware that many popular sauces contain gluten: salad dressings, soy sauce, barbecue sauce, gravy mixtures, marinades, and ketchup to name a few. Also, beware of most baked goods including cookies, cakes, muffins, pancakes, and waffles, and most pastas are made with gluten-containing grains. The same applies to snacks, chips, candy bars, granola bars, and pretzels. Take note also that many gluten-free foods may contain less fibre, be absorbed quickly and may, therefore, pose the danger of spikes in blood sugar.

QUINOA

Quinoa is an increasingly popular food in Western countries and found in the "ethnic" food section in supermarkets. It is more of a seed than a grain and is a relative of spinach and beets. It is considered a "nutritional powerhouse": high in plant protein, includes nine critical amino acids, and is packed with manganese, copper, and other vitamins and minerals.

It is, however, not a low-carb food. It carries a glycemic index of 53, in the middle of between the good and bad carb ranges. One cup yields more than 39 grams of carbohydrates, about eight grams of protein (twice the amount from white rice) and about five more grams of fibre compared to white rice. White rice yields 15 times the carbohydrates and 40 more calories compared to a cup of quinoa considered to be a healthier food choice. Quinoa fills you up faster, keeps you full overall longer, and therefore allows for smaller portion sizes thereby reducing food intake. The conclusion is that while quinoa takes on a similar texture to rice, the nutritional value is higher and more akin to its leafy vegetable relatives. All this explains the increasing popularity of quinoa.

THE ROLE OF FIBRE IN THE MANAGEMENT OF OBESITY

Fibre is of considerable dietary importance in the management of obesity. It slows the rate of digestion and, therefore, the rate of sugar absorption. Having to untangle the sugar from the fibres, so to speak, slows down the digestive process. Highly processed foods mean that very little fibre, if any, is left intact. Once isolated, the separated fibre exits the digestive system.

The quality of carbohydrates affects the level of cravings. Bad carbohydrates, such as highly processed carbs, create a craving for more bad carbohydrates; the individual eats more, and more is left for the deposit of fat.

Keep in mind that the simple carbohydrates lack both fibre and protein, both of which help to slow down digestion and balance sugar in the blood stream. The refining process strips these bad carbohydrates of their nutrient dense casings, leaving the simple carbohydrate chain.

For simple illustration, eating beans causes less hunger than potatoes; raw carrots cause less hunger than if cooked; eating whole fruit leads to less hunger than the same fruit pureed; drinking the juice only creates the highest level of hunger. There is a "glucose effect" since glucose is a form of energy constantly needed by the brain. Too low and levels lead to cravings for the carbohydrate fix. The brain detects hypoglycemia and reacts; hence the name, "reactive hypoglycemia."

It should be noted that acidic foods, such as lemon and vinegar, reduce the rate at which the stomach empties, thereby helping to control rising in blood sugar; dressing salads and vegetables with both has its dietary advantages.

Indications are that the human body evolved from a dietary pattern or ancestral nutritional landscape consuming large quantities of unprocessed plants. The recommended minimum adequate fibre intake approximates 30 g per day.

The general picture in North America is that about 97% of individuals get enough protein, a similar percentage not getting enough fibre—that is, about 25 g per day for women and 38 g for men. It is important to note that in the absence of an adequacy of fibre and the feeling of fullness, such as happens with the reduced fibre content of processed foods when calories are divorced from fibre, the internal signals is to ramp up food intake (and the calories) at the same time.

People talk a lot about the importance of fibre. There is a minimum knowledge base due to public health messaging about its nutritional importance. However, other questions arise. How knowledgeable are individuals about what fibre is and what are good sources? A serious paucity of knowledge may well abound. The individual dealing with an obesity issue must know that, by definition, fibre is only found in plants. It is totally absent in meat, dairy, and eggs, and it is definitely not being sourced by piling in junk food. Whole plant foods are the significant source of natural abundance. The data suggests that white bread, severely depleted of fibre, is in fact the number one source of fibre in the American diet and very likely much of the "developed" Western world.

Those of us who may be a little smug about our hearty Intake of fruits and vegetables need to realise that fruits and leafy veggies are the poorest whole-food sources of fibre. Why? Because they are 90 percent water. Root vegetables have about twice as much on a per weight basis, but the super-stars are whole plant foods in which dietary fibre is concentrated; whole grains and legumes, which include dried or canned beans, split peas, chickpeas and lentils.

An interesting article (*Women's World*, 2021) makes reference to "viscous fibre… as being a super fibre much more powerful than regular fibre… a great way to lose weight." It absorbs up to 50 times its weight in fluid. Water added creates a thick gel which becomes remarkably effective in reducing the production of fat storage hormones and facilitates the release of fat-burning compounds called butyrates. Reference is made to Canadian research indicating that 8 grams of this fibre sets up the recipient to "86% more ab flab and lose 73% more weight than if we skipped it." The suggestion is aim at about 20 grams of total fibre per day will guarantee at least about 10 grams of the viscous fibre.

GENERAL ADVANTAGES OF PLANT-BASED FOOD

Processed foods and animal products, loaded with fat, trans fat, and cholesterol, are found to be pro-inflammatory compared to the anti-inflammatory qualities of whole plant foods, such as fibre and phytonutrients. Pro-inflammatory diets are especially associated with abdominal obesity. It is known that fatty tissue actively secretes inflammatory chemicals into the blood stream and that obesity leads to systemic inflammation. The top five sources of saturated fat in a Western diet include cheeses, desserts (cake, ice cream), chicken, pork, and burgers.

It is useful to know the relationship between meat consumption and insulin levels, already discussed earlier in the text, in arriving at conclusions on dietary patterns to be pursued. Meat protein causes almost the same amount of insulin to be released as for pure sugar, my favourite "SOB" of weight management! It is reported that meat consumers have up to 50% higher insulin levels in their blood stream (Greger, 2019).

Research has shown that shifting persons from animal fats to plant fats, and without changing the quantity of dietary fat, leads to noticeable improvement in insulin sensitivity. Significant differences can be recorded in about 3 weeks.

The addition of egg whites, an animal product, to an ongoing plant-based dietary pattern has been shown to cause a 60% rise in insulin output in a matter of 4 days. More broadly speaking, meat consumption is associated with increased insulin levels, weight gain, and a higher risk of diabetes. Reportedly, a 5% substitution of plant protein for animal protein can decrease diabetes risk by 23%. Understandably, there is ongoing dialogue on the "meat-obesity connection" (Greger, 2019).

In essence, an increase in plant-based dietary intake leads to less insulin resistance and health improvement with respect to the numerous associated health challenges discussed earlier in the text. Australian research findings indicate that feeding individuals about the same number of calories and the same amount of fat, but switch over from meat and butter fat to plant-based olive oil, nuts, and avocados, can lead to nearly six more pounds of fat in a single month (Greger, 2019).

VEGANISM: THE MEANING OF "VEGAN" AND THE DIETARY ADVANTAGES

Dialogue on a diet largely or fully based on plant foods usually brings on the perspective of the individual being a vegan. Opinions on what dietary behaviour defines a person in this category varies.

Veganism is an indication of a person who abstains from the use of animal products, especially with respect to food consumption. Generally, meat is completely avoided, but there is likely to be some variation in dietary consumption as indicated above.

There are a few categories of veganism. A strict vegetarian is referred to as a "dietary vegan," one who eliminates meat, eggs, and dairy products; in essence, any industrial use of animal food. However, some persons who consider themselves vegan are criticized for consuming eggs and honey. A more extreme category opposes the use of animals in any aspect of life and for any purpose; such a person has been labelled as an "ethical" or "moral" vegan.

One presentation on the overall vegetarian spectrum lists the following:

Semi-Meatless: eats some meat, poultry and fish; milk, eggs, fruits vegetables, legumes, whole grains; avoids meat several times a week.

Pesco-Vegetarian: eats fish, milk, eggs, fruits, vegetables, legumes, whole grains. Avoids meat and poultry

Lacto-Ovo-Vegetarian: eats milk, eggs, fruit, vegetables, legumes, whole grains. Avoids meat, poultry and fish.

Vegan: avoids meat, dairy, fish, eggs, and sometimes other animal-derived foods, such as honey and gelatin.

NOTE: Indications are that any follower of a vegan-type diet will need to give attention to supplementary nutrient intake to ensure sustained good health. All four are recommended to consider a multivitamin, varying somewhat depending on the dominant food consumption pattern. Particular requirements may include iron, omega-3 fats, vitamin C, vitamin D, B12 supplements or B12-fortified foods, calcium, and zinc. Vitamin B12 occurs only in natural foods and is of special importance with respect to maintaining healthy nerve and blood cells and the making of DNA. Vitamin B12 deficiency can lead to fatigue and memory problems.

Vegans tend to have significantly less fat trapped in their muscle cells—a definite indication of less insulin resistance and lower insulin levels. The significant improvement in metabolic health arising from the indicated dietary shifts has even led to the suggestion that the said benefits may accompany an "intermittent vegan diet" in food consumption—that is, alternating between animal and plant protein choices (Greger, 2019).

Research findings are very encouraging to individuals considering a shift to a vegan-type lifestyle. Committed vegans for at least 5 years have shown a 26% less likelihood of dying from heart disease. An interesting indication is that individuals eating nuts more than 4 times a week suffer fewer than half as many heart attacks as persons who eat nuts less than once a week. Even semi-vegetarians have shown a 23% reduction in the relative risk of hypertension when compared to people who consume those items frequently. An even more striking research finding was that vegans who avoid animal products altogether showed a risk reduction of developing high blood pressure by as much as 75%. Compiled data for many studies indicate a 55% lower risk of developing high blood pressure for those who follow a vegan diet.

In general, vegetarian eating is associated with lowered risk of heart disease, keeping cholesterol level in check, improved blood pressure, a leaner body type, declining risk of diabetes, protection against cancer and a host of other diseases, and reduced living expenditure.

A plant-based diet has been shown to result in significant elimination of the deeper, more dangerous fat; a finding of major significance in choosing dietary staples when struggling with the battle of obesity.

SUMMARY

The decision to embark on a whole plant diet is clearly a trend which is receiving increased emphasis over time. In this chapter, it is made clear that a wide range of options exist for the decision maker. Plant-based food consumption has avid followers who range from just acceptance as the healthy way to eat to those who face a real struggle with extreme obesity. The broad spectrum of vegan consumption patterns tells the story.

The complete adoption of strictly plant-based diet can be somewhat of a drastic change compared to the traditional diet which includes animal-based foods in different forms. Also, it is reasonable to conclude that a vegan-type dietary focus on whole-plant-based foods has advantages when engaged in the struggle with obesity.

In summary, scientific research data has uncovered important reasons to support emphasis on plant-based diets. These include:

1. An abundance of antioxidants which slow the ageing process and hinder the development of cancer and heart disease;
2. The fibre advantage (whole grains, legumes, and fruit) which slows digestion, helps blood sugar control, satisfies the appetite, and promotes weight control;

3. The anti-inflammatory effects of unsaturated fats in olive oil, nuts, avocados, fish, and other selected food types which stave off heart disease.

On the basis of reported success, there is no doubt that embarking on a whole plant-based diet is a credible option for individuals with a concern about their level of obesity. In essence, if all other efforts fail and the obesity problem is of serious concern, both psychologically and in a real day-to-day sense, it does appear that this choice may well be a default option.

CHAPTER 9
EXERCISE PART 1: SELECTED GENERAL INFORMATION

EVERY INDIVIDUAL FACED with problems of weight management will need to understand the importance of exercise compared to all other initiatives under consideration in combatting this health challenge.

Most individuals have an overrated expectation of the importance of exercise, especially as compared to diet, in weight management. The overwhelming point of view is that incorporation of some measure of meaningful physical exercise on a sustained basis is absolutely necessary for effective weight management; more so if one is faced with the challenge of obesity.

The individual ought to be weary of the various adverts promising success in weight management by using a particular product; in particular, those which emphasise that success is achievable without having to make any lifestyle changes, including not having to pay any attention to an exercise component for sustainable results.

Given the apparent broad global participation, in particular, of walking as a form of exercise, Part 2 [Chapter 10] focuses on the core fundamentals relating to the importance of exercise in tackling the obesity problem. In essence, Parts 1 and 2, together, provide the reader with comprehensive information to provide guidance in formulating an exercise programme focussed on weight management and obesity.

CALORIE: ENERGY AND THE "BURN" IN EXERCISE

Any discussion on exercise brings attention to the concept of energy burn to achieve effective weight reduction. At this point, the term "calorie" comes to the fore. It cannot b e ignored in the presentation of information related to exercise.

As a reminder, calorie is a unit of heat or energy that raises heat of 1 gram of water by one degree Celsius. It illustrates what happens to the human body in any state of mobility, be it sedentary or at any range of intensity. Put simply, both the type and amount of food we eat determine how many calories are consumed eating a single food item or an entire meal.

The calorie burn comes with physical exercise and is applicable to any activity which consumes energy. Excess fat is burnt; it is important to develop a consciousness of the need to burn calories in the exercise process to use it as an effective tool in weight management. In essence, excess body fat is not wished away mentally; it has to be burned away! Bodily movement is a necessity.

EXERCISE AND ITS POSITIVE EFFECT
ON OUR ENERGY BALANCE

Let us look at what is known as the energy balance equation. This relates to the consumption and expenditure of energy with both sides being measured in calories.

Anyone who faces the issue of excess weight should remember: *Too little energy in or too much energy out leads to weight loss.*

Take a look at the equation:

Body fat = Calories IN (food, beverages) –
Calories OUT (metabolism, motion)

Therefore, what does not come out (burnt away) leaves you with the challenge of excess fat which stays on. Greger (2019) puts it more simply:

"Body Fat = Food + Beverages – Metabolism
– Exercise – Other Movement"

The "in" and "out" sides do not need to balance daily; however, if equalised, an individual is better able to sustain a healthy weight.

From a holistic point of view, balance is achieved when total calories consumed equals total calories used or burnt. It is affected by exercise and all forms of physical activity and also by body size and the amount of muscle and body fat present. One's genetics also has its effect.

So! If you are facing up to the challenge of obesity, anchor this simple fact in your subconscious: you can seriously determine what goes into your body, and therein lies a major aspect of the source of the fundamental difference in the outcome of your total effort towards achieving your weight management goal. Success is very much determined by how you manoeuvre your energy balance.

Exercise is clearly a key variable in the out portion of the formula. It is important that we understand how much exercise helps in tackling the obesity problem. In the context of energy burn, what does it take to make exercise work towards the goals of the obese individual? There are real surprises in what available information tells us.

In both Chapters 9 and 10, effective calorie burn is discussed in relation to levels of activity intensity and in the context of procedures for measuring individual achievement from a single workout routine. Comparative information with respect to walking as a mode of exercise is provided in Part 2.

TYPES OF EXERCISE

Varying core terms or types of exercise are available. The various alternative names reflect the nature of the physical activity. However, the major categories seem to be covered by aerobic, strength or resistance, and high intensity. Additional related terms encountered include resistance training, strength training, aerobic exercise, external resistance, and high intensity resistance.

These are discussed in some detail to ensure that the reader has some information to facilitate good decision-making. The individual, however, is obliged to seek guidance from the relevant experts in the field. Gym memberships are not necessarily cheap, but some formal tutoring in designing and pursuing exercise regimes can reduce the occurrence of serious injuries and lead to higher levels of success in achieving set goals. At the same time, gym-based programmes simply are not attractive for some individuals who, therefore, must seek alternative exercising routines to achieve successful weight management.

Metabolic AKA Strength or Resistance Training

Metabolic training is basically a form of exercise designed to improve muscular strength and fitness and build both muscle and endurance capacity. Increasing muscle tone is a process which requires more calories to maintain than fat. The body, therefore, burns more calories for daily upkeep even when sleeping.

Generally, the emphasis here is the use of compound exercises targeting multiple joints and muscles all at the same time. This pattern differs from isolated body building workouts which focus on specific muscle groups, one at a time, such as bicep curls. The multi-targeting effort (full body) stimulates more muscle fibres and supposedly has a hormonal effect which accomplishes faster muscle building and with a longer recovery effect, meaning that fat burning continues, possibly for as long as 36 hours.

This type of training is recommended for at least two to three times a week.

High Intensity Interval Training and Calorie Burn

"HIIT" is an abbreviation for high-intensity interval training.

We have already established that any exercise programme must pay attention to ways and means of achieving effective calorie burn. We also know exercise's limitations and, above all, consistent will power and time allocation are serious issues for successfully tackling the battle of the bulge. In this regard, the findings on the application of HIIT to your general fitness training, or more specifically to the struggle with excess fat, become significant.

It is a cardiovascular exercise strategy associated with what is known as "sprint" or "interval" training; that is, it alternates short periods of intense anaerobic exercise (short bursts of vigorous exercise) with less intense periods of recovery (low-intensity activity or rest). The principle here is that one can achieve burning the same total number of calories in a shorter time period. This is the expectation of a well-designed HIIT workout involving different exercises. It is especially efficient in its potential for increasing cardiorespiratory fitness.

The resistance aspect is accounted for by movement of the body against external resistance. The muscles contract against the resistance with the expectation of increases in strength, power, hypertrophy, and endurance. Hypertrophy is an increase and growth of muscle cells (muscle size) achieved through exercise, such as weight-lifting. The concept involves pushing the muscles to their limits through increased training volume (more sets and reps).

Resistance may be applied through strength exercises via free weights (dumbbells), weight machines, or the personal body weight of the partici-pant. Examples of the range of activity within this category include lifting weights, cycling, climbing stairs or hill walking, dance, use of resistance bands, push-ups, sit-ups, squats, bench press, lunges, and also heavy gar-dening (digging, lifting).

Two simple examples are:
- Squats or push-ups for 20 seconds and rest for 10 seconds
- Running in place for 60 seconds and rest for a few seconds

Overall findings caution anticipation of total outcome from this HIIT strategy over time. It would appear that there is moderate benefit in per-formance, in terms of "significant weight or body fat loss," as compared to standard engagement in continuous moderate intensity activity over a comparative period.

SIT [Sprint Interval Training] is another exercise strategy with a similar protocol; it also raises heart rate but maximises each movement to the point of feeling fatigued. It may use the same exercises as HIIT but with greater intensity and longer rest periods, such as using of jump squats instead of regular squats. An example of a 10-minute workout is jump squats or push-ups for 30 seconds followed by a 5-second rest period. The protocol is not recommended for early beginners.

The Tabata Workout

The Tabata workout fits within the HIIT regime. It is an effective workout designed with short, timed, high intensity intervals with short recovery periods. It is convenient for short available time periods. It consists of eight 20-second intervals of maximum high-intensity exercise, separated by 10-second periods of rest for 4 minutes. The challenges aim both aerobic and anaerobic systems in that it burns fat while boosting both endurance and cardiovascular performance; clearly not a routine for the faint-hearted! [Experience Life, October 2017]

Compared to HITT which has a more conservative effect on heart rate, 80 to 95 % of maximum heart rate, Tabaca aims to get heart rate above 100%

Cumulative findings are worthy of special attention. Weight loss is lasting. A 10% cortisol drop and 10% testosterone rise after an interval workout results in a hormone ratio which stimulates muscle build-up and a burning of belly fat as fuel. The improved midsection results tend to be more lasting.

Five main benefits of a HIIT programme include:
- Increased physical strength
- Increased weight loss
- Increased muscle mass which decreases with age
- Increased bone health: stronger bones, increased bone density with a reduced risk of fractures and related injuries
- Stabilization of joint flexibility; reduction of symptoms of arthritis

Strength or resistance training is reportedly good for all ages and levels of fitness, and is beneficial to individuals with a range of chronic health conditions including obesity and arthritis. Strength exercises reportedly help to prevent injury from an exercise regime by keeping weak muscles from becoming overpowered by stronger ones; this is very important, especially when engaged in active running routines.

There is some concern with respect to the underrating of resistance exercise for effective weight loss compared to longer, more stressful exercise routines. The idea seems to be that shorter workout periods with focussed targeting of movements can contribute to what is frequently referred to as "ageing backwards."

AEROBIC OR CARDIOVASCULAR EXERCISE

Aerobic exercise increases cardiovascular function by making the heart beat faster and increasing breathing and blood flow that brings oxygen quicker to the limbs. The overall effect, however, does not force the feeling of a need to rest. These exercises facilitate maximum fat-burning and heart-beating benefits, helping to burn fat more efficiently.

Aerobic exercise, such as swimming, walking, and jogging, raises heart rate and breathing for sustained periods. Aerobic exercises are very effective at impacting the intra-abdominal, visceral fat mentioned in Chapter 2.

In a general sense, walking is often the first choice of most individuals, and accessing its benefits are more likely to see sustained action in personal effort with continuity. As I have already indicated, walking is the focus of greater detail in Chapter 10

NOTES ON SELECTED COMMON EXERCISES

An individual in pursuit of effective weight management has a wide range of options available. Hereunder, selected information is presented on popular options which may be pursued by the individual seriously concerned about tackling the challenge of obesity.

Swimming

Swimming as a form of exercise has the advantage of working the entire body from head to toe. It allows for varying swimming patterns or strokes, each one focussing on different muscle groups of the body within a smooth watery environment, providing very gentle resistance.

It enables the use of most muscle groups while propelling the body through water, at the same time engaging the cardiovascular system: the heart and lungs. Among its many advantages:

- A possible option for individuals with various disabilities
- Significant reduction in joint pain and body stiffness
- Indications of being beneficial for persons with osteoarthritis, asthma, multiple sclerosis, dementia, and sleeping problems

- Acts like a mood booster and stress reducer
- Indications of many advantages similar to land-based exercises

Swimming is also very efficient at burning calories. For example, a 160-lb person will burn approximately 423 calories an hour swimming laps at a low or moderate pace, and 715 calories at a vigorous pace. For a 200-lb person, the figures are 528 and 982 respectively. Compare this with land-based activity and the 160-lb person loses 314 calories walking at 3.5 mph for 1 hour and 365 calories with elliptical training (treadmills, rowers, exercise bikes, jump rope). You can find more excellent information at www. fitnessvolt.com.

Indications are that swimming does not appear to be always very effective in the weight loss endeavour; there is strong indication, however, of having the potential to significantly boost appetite, increasing hunger much more than running and cycling. Swimmers tend to have more body fat than runners at the same level of physical activity. It appears that swimmers may well enjoy one half the risk of death compared to non-swimmers.

Cycling
Cycling is a form of exercise which has been shown to increase brain connectivity; at any intensity it, supposedly, corrects a depressed mood.

Yoga
Yoga is essentially based on lifting your own bodyweight and is executed through a series of what are called "poses." It is reportedly very effective in stress release.

Tai Chi
Tai chi is executed via a series of gentle movements which can be very deceptive with respect to their effectiveness on human health. Indications are strengthening of the back, abs, and the upper and lower body, and can be an effective form of pain release.

SEDENTARY LIFESTYLE (SITTING)

Let's take a peek at persons who spend a lot of their time sitting; say, a sedentary lifestyle. There can be vast differences in the accumulation of body fat between individuals consuming the same number of calories. The explanation lies in different patterns of cumulative movement and related energy expenditure.

.An overview of the literature indicates caution over how we overemphasise expectations on weight loss effect based on exercise alone. This has been labeled a kind of "myth" or common misconception in the field of obesity. There is a strong positive relationship between obesity and inactivity; however, to anchor down on exercise as the priority consideration is a big mistake.

Workplace routine patterns, such as sitting at a desk daily, will result in limited muscle movement and an inadequate blood flow supply. and it is suggested that a 15-minute mid-work stretching routine will improve both blood and nutrient flow to muscles and counter-attack discomfort and fatigue.

A similar recommendation based on research over at least 5 years is getting up every 30 minutes or standing for at least 9 minutes every hour. [The Zoomer Guide, 100 Years Strong,2022]. A recent report from Harvard Health points out that too many hours of sitting is linked to brain issues. Inactivity for more than 10 or more hours is associated with a higher risk of developing dementia at a later stage. Further analysis indicates the risk rising by 50% with 12 hours of inactivity and almost tripling at 15 hours [Harvard, 2023].

It is estimated that sitting more than 3 hours a day may be responsible for more than 400,000 deaths every year worldwide. Sitting has been referred to as the "new smoking."; more than 8 hours per day supposedly results in a life expectancy equal to people who smoke. A largescale study of 5000 women found that inactivity was more threatening than smoking cigarettes [Swap and Drop Diet, 2012]

A sedentary lifestyle puts the brakes on our metabolism. A shift from walking to sitting means that one's actual calorie burn is accompanied by a drop in calorie burn of about 33 %; from 3 per minute to 1 per minute.

Blood sugar and triglyceride levels rise while levels of good cholesterol [HDL.] fall. [Dr Ozz, 2020]

Reported research from USA, Norway and Sweden indicates that 8 to 35 minutes of moderate -to-vigorous physical activity [MVPA] a day led to risk of death plateauing at 11 minutes, so long as sedentary behaviour did not exceed 8.5 hours. [The Zoomer Guide, 2022]

Even sexual activity and calorie burn can be misunderstood. The calorie burn is much less than many may anticipate. [Greger, 2019]

All indications are that there is a relationship between dietary cravings and personal lifestyle movement habit. A sedentary lifestyle leads to a tendency towards a preference for fat- and calorie-rich foods while resisting carbohydrate-rich foods. Small amounts of exercise, such as a 2-mile daily walk, can reverse this preferential pattern.

When to Exercise: Timing

There is some variation in opinion on the matter of timing of exercise in relation to after or before a meal. There is a generalization that when done after a meal, the muscles can use stored material. Long- versus short-duration exercise and even differences in individual response are part of the discussion.

Sources of fuel used by the body are body fat (stored as glycerides) and carbohydrates (stored in the muscle and liver]); carbs are also available as blood sugar. Keep in mind that with respect to metabolic action (energy burn) the body has the ability to trade off between these two main sources, fat and carbohydrate; that is, one can exercise for hours with or without a recent meal.

Exercising on an empty stomach, referred to as a "fasted body," means that body fat is more readily targeted as a fuel source. In this regard, there is a suggestion that exercising at least 6 hours after the last meal may be advantageous. However, individual differences appear to be sufficient to disallow scientists concluding any general agreement that a fasting condition leads to greater fat loss over time. This also applies even to the HIIT pattern of exercise training.

Nevertheless, some sources state definitely that pre-meal exercise has definite advantages, such as at least 6 hours without food before breakfast, and that pre-breakfast walking has indicated an advantage of about 700 calories in fat loss; that is, more burning takes place. The explanation here is that the muscles dip into the body's energy storage for stuff to burn as fuel, reaching for some combination of glycogen and fat, both being stored materials. In this regard, it has been suggested that pre-breakfast exercise can burn as much as 18% of stored glycogen. An added advantage seems to derive from the fact that as glycogen storage decreases, the greater the sustained 24-hour fat loss.

There would seem to be some indications of improved performance with a meal before short duration aerobic exercise (including HIIT). Long-duration workouts, exceeding 1 hour and requiring endurance, also seem to benefit from a pre-exercise meal consisting mostly of carbohydrates as long as 3 to 4 hours before the workout. Greater agreement appears to be on having a post workout meal to aid muscle recovery, especially if the exercise was pre-fasted.

Research also indicates a relationship between the timing of exercise and memory power. The results favour exercise after a future memory retrieval task. Better recall and more desirable activation of areas of the brain related to information retrieval resulted from exercise approximately four hours after exposure to the memory task. [Time, 2019]

Diabetics and Timing

There is additional information of relevance to diabetics. Individuals affected by elevated blood sugars are reported to derive benefits from post meal exercise with respect to the lowering of the readings.

Even a leisurely 20-minute stroll at about 2–3 mph demonstrates a positive blunting of sugar spikes by about 30%. This group of individuals, therefore, can claim benefits for both pre- and post-meal exercise regimes, possibly with advantages on the post-meal side. It is indicated that even a 10-minute walk makes a difference after any meal, dinner or breakfast being the priority choices.

Blood sugar elevation in the blood stream commences 20 minutes after the first bite and peaks at about 1 hour later. Greger[2019] suggests that diabetics and prediabetics start exercising 30 minute safter the start of a meal and ideally go for an hour to completely straddle the blood sugar peak.

APPETITE AND EXERCISE: NET GAIN OR LOSS OF WEIGHT

There is what one may call an appetite effect associated with exercise to be guarded against. Expending energy through exercise can dispose an individual to becoming hungry physiologically and to consume more food. The body does not like to be in deficit with respect to its fat storage; this means there is a possibility of the body attempting compensation by increased calorie intake (increased appetite) over time to match calorie expenditure from exercise. This makes significant weight loss difficult but not impossible; net loss in body fat must be monitored to check on progress.

If one has an uncontrollable appetite which hinders weight control management, the real objective is to get to a food-intake-cum-exercise-burn threshold, where the exercise activity outpaces the appetite. Success will only be achieved if one can keep calorie intake below calorie expenditure; energy balance again!

One cannot lose sight of the matter of calories in determining expectations from an exercise regime.

Calories in = Calories out.

In essence, all calories are not the same; this being so, one ought not to expect a 500-calorie walk to offset the negative health effect of a 500-calorie meal on the "in" side.

UTILISING THE AFTER-BURN EFFECT OF EFFICIENT EXERCISE

When considering the benefits of exercise, it is worth being aware of the added edge, referred to as an "afterburn effect" or excess post-exercise oxygen consumption (EPOC). The core contribution of exercise in dealing with the obesity challenge is that it revs up the metabolic rate of the individual; it burns!

After exercise, there is the matter of the resting metabolic rate. As much as a 5%–10% increase is experienced as an after effect. To illustrate its significance, consider the 150 calories burnt with a brisk half-hour walk. A 7% boost for the subsequent 36 hours means an added EPOC effect of burning an additional 170 calories. This added effect can be experienced for up to 48 hours after a single bout of exercise.

Pritikin (1998) provides a unique and impacting explanation on the relationship between exercise and burning off fat:

1. The body stores about 1500 calories of energy from carbohydrates in muscles and liver (call it the carbohydrate fuel tank)
2. Lean-bodied persons store about 66 times this amount as fat
3. Overweight persons store about 133 to 200 times the amount
4. This means that the amount of fat stored in body tissue exceeds considerably the amount of carbohydrate stored
5. The body burns a fuel mix of approximately 50% of each type; i.e., the fuel tank versus fat storage
6. The body relies almost exclusively on carbohydrates (not fat) as fuel for brain function and rapid physical action
7. This means that putting a dent in the fat reserves is no easy task and that there is a constant requirement to renew the carbohydrate-supplied fuel from the muscle/liver tank for the purpose at (f) above. Comparatively speaking, the demand from the fat tank pales in size. There is, inevitably, a constant depletion of the carbohydrate storage tank (a lowering of carbohydrate reserves) and, therefore, a greater demand on the body to consume more carbohydrate rich foods. This leads to a kind of forced dietary change!

In essence, research (Pritikin, 1998) shows that calorie consumption associated with exercise is primarily from carbohydrates, intake increasing with activity accompanied by a reduction in weight:

> Food preferences are changed by exercise... if you don't exercise, your body will limit the amount of carbohydrate foods you can safely eat... if you discipline yourself to eat a high carbohydrate diet but don't exercise enough, the excess carbohydrates you eat can be converted to triglycerides or fats in your liver and then flood your bloodstream with tiny globules of fat. Elevated i.e. increased levels of triglycerides can lower

high-density lipoproteins, or HDLs, the "good" cholesterol that reduces your risk of heart disease.

MUSCLE TYPE AND CALORIE BURN

Success at gaining body muscle mass through exercise also carries advantages in the battle against fat loss. Exercise boosts metabolic rate (Greger, 2019).

Increased muscle mass burns more calories and raises the basic metabolic rate (BMR), the amount of energy (calories) needed to keep the body functioning while at rest. This basal metabolism is usually the largest component of a person's total caloric needs in order to sustain organ function.

According to Shin Otake [www.maxworkouts.com] there is a connection of the body's nervous system to weight loss and muscle building. Total energy expenditure must be embedded in the personal psyche in the battle with fat loss. Aim to increase the BMR. Trigger the afterburn effect that will last for hours.

Supposedly, for every pound of muscle added to the body, an additional 50 calories per day are burnt while the body is at rest. For example, add 2 lb of body muscle and burn approximately an additional 700 calories per week. This means that a change in body composition leads to a loss of an additional 12 lb of fat in a year.

In the context of diet, the recommendation is that small, dispersed, and orderly meal consumption patterns bring on a higher BMR and increased fat loss.

The challenge, therefore, is that fat reduction and replacement on arms, under chin, leg muscles, and belly helps with extra fat burn even when just sitting around.

EXERCISE AND AGEING

The ability to move about generally deteriorates with ageing and it is therefore necessary to keep this phenomenon in mind when assessing and planning physical activity for older people. Older individuals leading a sedentary lifestyle lose 30%–40% of the stock of fibres in their muscle by age 80. With decreased movement, metabolism slows down and the fibres shrink and atrophy. Ageing generally means less responsiveness to exercise.

Strength training in later years is aiming at achieving regrowth and revitalisation of atrophied fibres.

Ageing is accompanied by increased cortisol levels and decreasing levels of testosterone; the result is a breaking down of lean muscle tissue and increased fat storage in the midsection. This development calls for caution in extreme exercise workouts since there is a build-up of cortisol levels which hinders the loss of stubborn fat.

One interesting article I encountered on difficulty in losing fat refers to "fascia" tissue which envelops every muscle, blood vessel, nerve, organ, and bone, and is generally pliable and flexible, facilitating internal movement. With ageing comes significant changes. Underused muscles, poor posture, and inflammation lead to scar tissue and an obstructive, binding effect: muscles becoming short, stiff, dysfunctional, weak, and withered. Exercise and movement, in general, can become uncomfortable and can be accompanied by pain, tension, and restricted blood flow. This condition relates to a decrease in oxygen supply which is necessary for the breaking down of fat; slowed metabolism hampers the body's capacity to burn fat, and there is impairment of the capacity to build and retain lean muscle. Excessive weight creeps up and it becomes all but impossible to lose weight.

Restricted, sticky, tight fascia affect the shape of our bodies and can contribute to that look of false belly fat and the appearance of cellulite with the dimpled look. The situation is supposedly corrected by diet and targeted massage which facilitate blood flow and a refiring of fat burn. The remedy seems to be smoothening out or loosening of the fascia resulting in increased muscle strength and tone with stubborn fat and cellulite vanishing.

The literature indicates that it is incorrect to believe that muscle cannot be gained past one's 60th birthday; indications are that even up to the 70th birthday, muscle building achievement can match success equivalent to individuals in their 40s.

Resistance or strength training is good for all ages and for a range of conditions related to obesity and arthritis. This type of exercise helps to prevent the natural loss of lean muscle which accompanies ageing.

There is the additional advantage derived from the fact that muscles at any age lead to a tighter, slimmer body and will facilitate the burning of more calories both at work and at rest. Increasingly, the data suggests that nearly everyone, including older persons, benefit from exercise. A Harvard study (2019) demonstrated that older adults performing the minimum recommended weekly exercise (even if relatively inactive in younger years) lived longer and with a 24% lower risk of dying from any cause during a 12-year period.

In large measure, many available activity monitors have been developed for young and middle-aged people who have higher physical performance than older adults. It has been suggested, therefore, that these monitors may underestimate actual levels of exertion in the activity of older adults.

As we age, declining cognitive function is demonstrated by well-known "senior moments" of not remembering simple things, increased reaction time, and even depression. There is high-quality evidence that exercise activity has many favourable benefits in the golden years. In this regard, exercise has been referred to as a non-pharmacological strategy to mitigate the deleterious effects of ageing on brain health, in some respects women benefitting more than men. Physical exercise reportedly induces structural plasticity in the human brain, thereby enhancing cognitive functions. Moderate intensity and frequency are recommended with programmes being personalised for maximum benefit.

For aged individuals and others who have a highly sedentary lifestyle, the internet carries information on simple exercise regimes designed for execution from a sitting position. Reportedly, people who simply "move a lot" during the day reduce the risk of early death by 30 %. [Oaklander,2016]

It is of interest to note that research further indicates exercise in the latter years affecting depression positively and even countering a tendency towards emotional and excess eating.

Fitness and Virtual Reality

The entry of Virtual Reality [VR] into the realm of exercise heralds new and exciting dimensions The integration of exercise and physical fitness into game development programmes is relatively new. and allows participants to enjoy the "cool effects" of the technology using headsets and the accompanying "cool" technology. The workouts are in the form of games and participants must move around to achieve selected goals. The resulting "gamercising' or VR" exergaming" is an emersive experience which requires a minimum level of balance control and facilitates hand-eye coordination and flexibility; indications of slowing age-related cognitive decline as related to Alzheimer disease and other dementias. Some programmes point to working well for seniors, for example Oculus and Rendever Fit. A range of realistic activity and imaginary engagement in different geographical spaces are indicated. [Cox, 2023]

SLEEP AND EXERCISE: SYNERGY WITH WEIGHT ACCUMULATION

An insufficiency of good, deep sleep can affect considerably our struggle with effective weight maintenance. Sleep has a symbiotic relationship with exercise and has been referred to as the foundation of health; it enhances the quality of life. The exercise-sleep combination has been researched and it is clear that moderate to vigorous exercise, such as walking, swimming, and yoga, do improve sleep quality the same night by reducing the time it takes to fall asleep and also decreasing the number of sleep interruptions experienced during the night.

A good night's sleep provides a refreshed and alert wake-up and exercise. The healthy individual needs enough of two different types of sleep: REM and non-REM types. Both are important.

There is a reference to the parasympathetic nervous system (PNS) or "rest and digest" system. The vagus nerve, one of the longest and most important nerves in the body, is important in the control of many crucial functions. In this regard, it has been regarded as the "information highway" between the brain and gut, and apparently can affect everything including mood, stress levels, digestion, heart rate, and immune response. A stimulated vagus nerve enables an individual to enter into the sleep process to a level of winding down which facilitates achieving a restorative state necessary for tissue repair and clearance of waste products, including toxins and waste proteins built up in the brain during the day. Inadequate sleep prevents the effective flushing out of the accumulated toxins.

Sleep deprivation may be occasional or in a chronic pattern for the individual, the adequate amount varying considerably between 6 and 9 hours of "shut eye." Chronic sleep deprivation has a major impact on personal health, the person experiencing both physical and mental symptoms. Cognitive performance (memory and motivation), effect on mood (effect on brain chemistry and hormones) and anxiety (stressful thoughts keeping you awake), increased sadness and depression, impaired ability to remain focussed—a wide range of tell-tale symptoms.

Generally, it appears that afternoon exercising brings on the best quality sleep; it is accompanied by a decline in adrenaline, heart rate, and body temperature, all of which facilitate sleep a few hours later. Moderate aerobic exercise increases the amount of "slow wave" sleep (SWS) experienced. SWS is called Phase 3 sleep, the deepest phase of non-rapid eye movement. Dreaming and sleep walking goes with this phase. It is also an important phase for memory consolidation.

There is a parallel relationship between sleep deprivation and weight gain due to the disruption of the hormones which regulate appetite, ghrelin, and leptin. Reported indications are that people eat an average an extra 300 to 384 calories per day as a result of sleep deprivation, thus leading to the scale effect, so to speak.

The effects on digestion relate to stimulating digestive enzymes and other digestive functions. The relationship between a healthy gut, good health, and problems of obesity receives considerable attention later on.

Deep, uninterrupted sleep also helps to maintain healthy levels of two important chemicals in metabolic function: melatonin and serotonin. Serotonin is a chemical that carries messages between nerve cells in the brain and throughout the body. It plays a key role in many body functions including mood, sleep, social behaviour, pain sensation, digestion, blood clotting, breathing, bladder control, and sexual desire. It is the precursor to melatonin: it becomes converted to the latter in darkness only. Approximately 95% of the body's supply is in the gut; an adequate supply being dependent upon a healthy gut. Symptoms of serotonin deficiency include seasonal and chronic depression, insomnia and sleep cycle disturbances, weight gain and carbohydrate cravings, chronic pain and muscle pain, and alcohol abuse.

Melatonin is a hormone produced in the brain and is necessary for regulating the sleep-wake cycle as well as our immune system. It helps with the control of our circadian rhythms (our 24-hour internal clock) and, therefore, our quality of sleep. It is a popular over the counter purchase for insomnia; however, there appears to be a scarcity of compelling research data on the advisability of this practice. My personal experience with over the counter purchase has not been very positive.

Meditation or controlled breathing are popular exercises that provide a calming transition for bedtime. It clears the mind of distracting thoughts while controlled breathing slows the heart and relaxes the body. In addition, these mental exercises can release relaxing hormones, reduce cortisol, and increase natural melatonin levels which facilitate more restful sleep.

The U.S. National Sleep Foundation recommends 7 to 9 hours of sleep per night for adults. Unfortunately, indications are that one in three adults get less than this amount resulting in build-up of "sleep debt"; the consequences register in both body and mind. Regretfully, I can testify to be a victim of this misfortune: diagnosed sleep apnea, affecting capacity to function during the day and so forth.

Sleep deprivation must not be underestimated in the struggle with obesity. My personal experience with diagnosis and treatment by a physiatrist brought home this reality to me on a personal basis. I was informed that the pain, sometimes quite extreme, I was experiencing across my waist resulted from a lack of serotonin due to inadequate sleep. In essence, my pathway to the termination of back pain focussed successfully on facilitating improved quantity of sleep, and including the supply of serotonin.

Seratonin is one of the "happy " hormones; others include oxytocin and dopamine. It works as a neurotransmitter relaying signals across the nervous system helping to regulate mood and other behavioral activity, including sleep. [www.sciencedirect.com]

Vaccariello (2012) points to important additional research results related to inadequate sleep and human health on a daily basis:

> Sleeping less than 6 hours per night can increase one's risk of developing diabetes as much as 30 percent because of the body's impaired ability to regulate blood sugar. Dieters who got 8½ hours of sleep on a nightly basis lost 56 percent more body fat compared to individuals on the same diet but only 5½ hours sleep per night.

Research allowing five hours a night sleep for 68,000 women by Harvard Medical School indicated a 32 percent greater likelihood of gaining 30 pounds or more as they get older, compared to women whose sleep regime was regularly 7 hours or more. [Sleep and Drop,2012]

The sleep deprivation admonition is so serious that it is suggested to avoid flipping on night switches when making bathroom visits or engaging in any temporary activity since one burst of brightness can temporarily suppress melatonin production; use of a flashlight is suggested. In countries which follow daylight saving time, the "lost hour" of sleep at change over each spring is accompanied by heart attacks shooting up by about 5% (Beil, 2011).

The Harvard Medical School (2020) recommends the practice of good sleep hygiene: "use the bedroom only for sleeping and sex, not for computing work, television watching or other activities." It is advocated that TV be banished from the bedroom.

IMPORTANCE OF HYDRATION AND EFFECTIVE WEIGHT LOSS

There is a general recommendation that for maximum effectiveness an exercise programme must ensure attention to adequate hydration (drinking enough water). For example, one recommendation before a morning run is to ensure having about 500 ml of water 30 to 60 minutes before starting the run.

Proper exercising should result in sweating. Failure to pay attention to adequate water intake makes weight loss much more difficult. Water in the human body ranges between 50% and 75% and is relevant to almost every biological body function.

Inadequate hydration causes a slowing down of metabolic activity; it affects both body temperature and productive muscle performance when exercising.

Indications are that the more you sweat, the more water you need. Depending on the exercise regime, half a glass of water at 10- to 15-minute intervals is advisable to replace fluid lost through sweating. Adequate water intake is also regarded as important in reducing the risk of injuries since it helps to maintain adequate lubrication of muscles and joints.

Adequate hydration has been referred to "as the key to making every weight loss diet successful." It is relevant to maintaining blood volume balance.

Drinking water increases the number of calories burned; it is known as "resting energy expenditure," referred to earlier in the chapter. In the case of adults, it is reported that within 10 minutes of drinking water, energy expenditure increases by 24%–30% and that the effect is sustained for as long as 1 hour. Increased water consumption by 1.5 litres per day could burn an extra 17,400 calories (5 lb) in 1 year.

An average recommendation is to aim for 2–2.5 litres (8 to 10 glasses) of water per day to avoid dehydration. Dehydration can cause fatigue and dizziness; energy levels drop and a diminishing of the feeling to exercise. Good water intake aids in maintaining focus, alertness, and a general feeling of being energised.

CORE MUSCLES: SOME FUNDAMENTALS

I have concluded that it is important to be aware of some minimal critical information with respect to what is routinely referred to as the "core": the need to pay attention to strengthening the core.

Knowing the muscles that make up the core and understanding their contribution to core coordination are important. At the top of the core sits the diaphragm, a dome-shaped sheet of muscle that plays a vital role in the breathing process. At the bottom lies the pelvic floor, a hammock of three muscle layers stretching from the tailbone to the pubic bone. This basic frame, together with other important muscles, connects the rib cage and pelvis. All together, they form what is referred to as a "three-dimensional canister" of muscles, bones, and other tissues that wraps around the body from front to back.

The core concept becomes clear; it is much more than the imagery of a healthy looking six pack abdominals. The core functions in a wholistic manner and the important point is that any weak sections negatively affect overall core performance. Proper positioning of the ribs and pelvis together with optimal functioning of the diaphragm and abdominal muscles are critical while pursuing a range of physical activities, including walking, running, exercising, and playing sports. With a strong, well-integrated core, these activities become easier, more enjoyable, and are performed with less risk. In addition, a strong core effectively optimises training sessions and allows for faster recovery time.

A weak or uncoordinated core with muscles not working together can lead to injury, impeded performance, back and joint pain, incontinence, and sexual dysfunction.

According to Lieberman,2020 :

> "All bodily movement, in every conceivable direction, originates in the core, and to strengthen it is to guard against injury, improve the body's functionality and build fitness from the inside out."

Building the core involves the proper application of breathing, positioning, and strengthening activity. Success in any physical endeavour depends on a strong and well-coordinated core—one that integrates muscular strength, control, mobility and breathing from the inside out."

STRETCHING

I consider it prudent to provide some information in this chapter on stretching. It does appear that many individuals embark on exercising initiatives because of weight concerns or perhaps simply an increased interest in general health, but without any understanding of the significance of stretching as part of an intended programme of activity.

"You're not done until you've stretched" is a common saying; stretching is the way to end your exercise session.

There are recommendations on stretching both before and after physical exercise. Muscles should be warmed up before stretching commences. After an exercise programme, they are already warm. Varying types and combinations of stretches are included in recommendations. Take note that yoga and pilates are recommended to achieve the same effects.

Stretching increases range of movement and helps to tone muscles. Before the exercise routine, stretching advantages relate to reduced soreness and the prevention of injury to muscles. It is considered essential after a strenuous workout and is recommended to be a part of a balanced programme, being given the same importance as inclusion of strength or vascular training.

Indications are that a 30 minute whole-body stretch 5 days a week is more effective at reducing blood pressure in older adults with hypertension compared to brisk walking for the same period. [The Zoomer Guide ,2022

Stretching is also part of an effective cool-down routine. Benefits of post routine or "cooling down" stretching include improved blood circulation; a cooling down of body temperature with assistance for lowering heart beat to facilitate a return to normalcy; preventing dizziness as it stops blood from suddenly pouring into hands and feet and facilitates wider body circulation; assisting muscle relaxation and enhancing flexibility and range; removal of waste from muscle tissue and faster recovery as it breaks the release of lactic acid which takes place during workout; and reducing the chances of muscle cramps and stiffness. Unstretched muscles remain constricted and tight, and there is a reduction in use from full capacity. Stretching also aids maintenance, decreases the risk of injury, promotes good posture, increases muscular coordination and functional mobility, and improves synchronization. It also enhances mental clarity and mind-body coordination beyond the muscles; there are indications of a positive effect on harmony of mood relaxation and stress relief.

A cautionary recommendation is to obtain coaching guidance where necessary; an alternative is to seek information on the topic and practice with caution and discipline.

Categorised stretch types include names such as quadriceps, chest, hamstring, hip, torso, inner thigh, marching, roll up, cat, cow, and so forth. This allows the individual to consider which group or combination of types to apply to an exercise programme—most likely based upon personal goals and preferences in application.

Five interesting stretches described in Dr. Oz's handy publication (2020) include the following::

Reaching for the sky, Calf Stretch, Hip Opener, Hamstring Easer and Quad Stretch.

With respect to achieving post-routine cooling down, the simplest way may be to proceed to a slower- or lower-intensity version of the exercise being performed.

Functional fitness is meant to convey someone having the combination of strength and agility to pursue daily life with relative ease. The types of exercise that promote functional fitness are primarily stretches together with crunches and other resistance type exercises. These exercises increase core body strength, flexibility, balance, and coordination together with improved posture.

GENERAL TIPS FOR AN EFFECTIVE EXERCISE PROGRAMME IN THE MANAGEMENT OF OBESITY

Finally, here are some tips various individuals offer to help make your exercise regime a success.

Balance Your Protein. While it is said to be useful to have a bit of protein after a workout in order to assist muscle repair and growth, avoid excess intake because what is not used up will be stored as fat, defeating the purpose of the exercise programme; 2% plain yogurt is one recommendation for this purpose.

The use of whey protein in combination with exercise is also reported to have a beneficial effect on testosterone levels; 15 g raising the hormone level by 25% for 48 hours, converting amino acids into muscle-building protein and achieving improved metabolism. Use of a whey shake after a workout has been shown to double fat loss and boost muscle gain by 63%.

Be Consistent. Focus on being consistent with your programmed schedule of exercise, whatever the type selected.

Fuelling Up Before Your Workout Can Help Performance. A carb-rich snack can make the workout better and can increase fat burning during the exercise; some individuals consume an apple or a plum, apparently best taken within 60 minutes of a serious endurance workout. A small protein and fruit smoothie is an alternative.

Don't Forget Breakfast. Prior to a challenging morning workout, such as hill climbing or lasting at least 90 minutes, performance can be enhanced by having breakfast (avoiding high fat or high fibre) preferably 2 to 3 hours before starting. Under average conditions, it is said that exercising on an empty stomach facilitates burning fat as the fuel; however, this condition is not considered as a prerequisite.

Challenge Your Muscles. If the performance of the routine, such as reps, is too easy, rev up the challenge. For illustration, a person with 150-lb bodyweight who increases the treadmill speed from 5 to 6 mph will boost calorie burn by 25%.

Do Not Underestimate the Importance of Recovery and Rest. Relaxation time between the challenging sweat sessions is important; if not, the stress hormone cortisol is released and there is a boost to fat storage and appetite for food.

Vary Your Exercises. Mix up the exercise routines so as to vary the muscles targeted in execution. One can even mix different types of exercise in order to boost personal enjoyment and minimise boredom. The mixture can include variation between consecutive days of cardiovascular (aka respiratory) strength training and flexibility exercises. This becomes important if one is not seeing results; small changes can give the body a jump start.

Do Not Underestimate the Use of a Personal Trainer. Even if consulted for only a few times at the start of an exercise programme, a personal trainer can be invaluable. They can show you how to use gym equipment properly; guide on hydration, sequence of selected activities, and repetitions; and advise on designing, executing, and adjusting the programme. Many elements contribute to the rate of personal progress and affect desired outcomes in the long run.

Try "Exercise Snacks." There is the question of how much exercise is necessary! Indications are that very long periods of aggressive activity, such as pumping iron, are not the only way to achieve one's goals. The evidence suggests that "exercise snacks" (Rheaume, 2023) (brief bouts of strength-training activities) can be very effective. Starters may do as little as little as 5 minutes twice daily of strength building movement and be as effective as lengthy periods in a gym. Use of a chair for balance followed by gradually incorporating weights, resistance bands, and light equipment can maintain effectively challenging "snack" sessions. A simple example may be:

- Squats: 60 seconds

- Standing calf raises: 60 seconds
- Push-ups: 60 seconds
- Plank: 60 seconds
- Stair climbing or on the spot jogging or skipping rope: 60 seconds

SUMMARY

The reader is reminded that Part 2 to this chapter includes a special presentation on walking, the most popular form of exercise.

While caution is indicated with respect to one's expectations of weight loss benefits to be gained from exercise alone, there is a clear indication of considerable overall health benefits of physical activity. Here is a brief listing of concluded good results.

Increased fitness will reduce the risk of breast cancer, colon cancer, hypertension, diabetes, gallstones, heart disease, and stroke. Exercise is medicine: it can improve insulin sensitivity for up to 17 hours and can be used to treat pre-diabetes, coronary heart situations, and stroke. Aerobic exercise over about 13 weeks, 30–60 minutes a day, can lead to fat loss.

In the search for results from exercise regimes, we are reminded that numbers on a scale may not reveal the full story of success. For example, obese diabetics in a research trial did not achieve significant loss in weight, but! there was a loss of about 8 lb of body fat while they gained an almost equivalent amount of lean body mass or muscle.

Let's take note of what is revealed about our most dangerous fat: the visceral fat slithering around our internal abdominal organs. Exercise has been proven to get rid of about 6% of visceral fat levels, apparently demonstrating better results than caloric restriction in this regard. It is quite interesting to find out that abdominal exercises alone, including stomach crunches, in spite of the optics in various advertising media, are not as effective as one may think in the reduction of waistlines.

It is suggested that the secret to weight loss through exercise may be sheer volume: at least 300 minutes a week to achieve appreciable fat loss. Waist line reduction is by no means an easy task and it is estimated to take as much as 3 hours of aerobic exercise a week over 3 months to take off an inch off our waist line.

Belittle not such an achievement! A medical, abdominal cross sectional review may reveal removal of 5 square inches of visceral belly fat. For effective fat removal from the toughest body locations housing the worst kind of fat, it is indicated that aerobic exercise has an edge over resistance training.

In reality, the fundamental to be remembered is that the "calorie deficits" referred to above have to get bigger so that the body tries to keep up by making withdrawals from one's body total fat. Keep calorie intake below calorie expenditure. Only significant amounts of exercise can cause significant weight loss.

Mere knowledge of the potential is not enough to achieve one's target objective in weight management. This information drives home an important point for each and every individual engaged in the battle of the bulge. Ultimately, the lesson to be learnt is that it takes a lot of work, indeed a lot of effort to achieve meaningful weight management. Exercise, like diet, only works if you actually do it.

One has to be aware of cumulative findings under different circumstances—what, when, where, and how with respect to making a determination on the nature of an exercise regime: its selection and execution. The individual must understand and accept that there must be a commitment to exercise regularly, beyond one's usual level of exertion. Only limited success can be achieved with low doses of prescribed exercise.

Even a 1,000-calorie exercise burn a day may lead to only a loss of about 1 lb in a week. Once again, fat loss through exercise alone is not a walk in the park, I may add, nor perhaps a casual hike up a gentle slope.

Nevertheless, exercise burns fat and weight is lost; also, because it helps to reorient food preferences, exercise appears to facilitate the best chance to keep off the weight lost in the process.

The American College of Sports Medicine has shown that exercise lowers the risk of stroke by 27%, reduces the incidence of diabetes and breast cancer by 50%, the incidence of high blood pressure and Alzheimer's by 40%, and colon cancer by 60%.

The U.S. National Academy of Medicine recommends a minimum of 1 hour exercise per day based on the habits of normal-weight people. Outside of this, the overwhelming recommendation for an exercise regime is 60–90 minutes per day of moderate exercise. It would seem that most individuals never achieve such targets and that less than 3% achieve as much as half an hour per day. Personally, it took me many months to get close to attempting the 1-hour recommendation for 3–5 days per week. A popular minimum recommendation is 300 minutes per week in order to achieve appreciable fat loss. Sheer volume is important.

There is also the challenge of the newcomer or loner trying to find guidance on a choice of exercise regime. There is a plethora of advertising offers from so-called "core exercisers and spin class junkies" all offering to fix your core and change bodies, using sweet sounding "protocols" and unique packages. Good people are misled by personal trainers, magazine articles, and late-night infomercials.

Older people, especially seniors, have an even more daunting task: remaining conscious of the need to avoid injury and save their money, especially when tempted to participate in exercise activity aimed at the silent desire to reverse the ageing process.

Clearly the benefits of exercise are expected to be good based upon any exercise regime, in and by itself. However, keep in mind that an individual has so much more control over the "calories in" side of the equation, compared to the "calories out." Your first order of business is to manage what you put in your mouth.

In a general sense, it is recommended that men over 45 and women over 55, especially if there are indications of health issues, such as diabetes, chest pains, dizziness, or shortness of breadth, should check with health professionals before embarking on any exercise regime.

Finally, let me end this section with a fundamental lesson in weight management. You are reminded to tame your expectations for success based only on exercise.

CHAPTER 10
EXERCISE PART 2: WALKING: A POPULAR FORM OF EXERCISE FOR ALL AGES

WALKING IS ONE of the most popular forms of exercise worldwide. It is the type of activity that comes to the fore in the aerobic or cardio category as described in Part 1 of the comprehensive presentation on exercise. It stands out as a low-impact, high-benefit, effective option in weight loss management. Active involvement does not require expensive equipment or any special skill, and it is said to have the lowest "quit rate" of any type of exercise.

Walking and strength training represent a dynamic duo, referred to as a "two in one workout" in the fitness world; for example, a 20-minute walk followed by 5 minutes strength training can replace 30 minutes of walking only. Both efficiency and effectiveness are projected. Together, they help to prevent injuries, slow down age-related body mass loss, and ensure a sustained amount of exercise without a burn-out effect, and, in the process, deliver a low-stress endurance boost to heart, lungs, and muscle.

A simple format is walking combined with weights (dumbbells), such as incorporating weights while you walk. This workout calls for choice of weights, such as would fatigue the muscles but are sustainable for the workout; also, positioning is important.

Numerous illustrations project the gains derived from walking under different conditions: how much is adequate, how many steps within a stated time period are sufficient for effective exercise, the pace of walking, length of time, intensity of effort, and variation with body weight.

NUMBER OF STEPS

To achieve fitness and weight loss, 10,000 steps in any single day is frequently suggested as a starting target to achieve visible results. The amount of time spent in achieving the target is by no means insignificant. For example, achieving this target within about an hour in any one day approximates walking about 5 miles. Depending on body weight, this achieves a burn of about 250–600 calories. It is not an easy task since the average relatively inactive person takes about 3,000 steps or less each day within a house.

A pedometer or the numerous apps on cell phones monitor movement of body over space; they allow us to approximate steps per mile and calories burned. An individual can log in at various threshold goals, such as 7,000–10,500, to achieve a targeted number of steps per day. It is also possible to generate personal walking plans geared to targeted weight loss indicators on your mobile phone.

Take note that the average daily household stepping achievement (3,000 steps), combined with a minimum targeted walking plan of 4500 to 5000 steps, gets you quite close (about 8,000) to the recommended daily target for good health. In the absence of wearing a pedometer at all times, I have found it useful to know the approximate number of steps used to traverse identified distances (by landmark) in the popular or preferred walking areas.

The Swat and Drop diet book gives us some interesting guidelines on number of steps to be take for effective weight loss. Interval training with its short bursts of harder effort is highly recommended. The Metabolic Equivalent of Task [MET] is discussed. One MET is the equivalent of burning 1 calorie per kilogram of body weight per hour; for example, body weight of 180 pounds [81 kg] means burning 81 calories per hour.

Maximum fat burn requires a minimum intensity of 3 METs per hour. Achieving this target is estimated at 100 steps per minute [spm]. Research indicates that interval training regularly yields better results compared to one speed workouts. [Swap and Drop, 2012]

Here are some interesting crude projections for aiding achievement of stepping goals on the basis of day-to-day living:

- A brisk 15-minute walk at any time, such as on the way to work, walking the dog, or a mid-morning neighbourly walk can gain at least 1,000 to 1,200 steps.
- Going to a bathroom one floor up or down can gain about 300 steps.
- Strolling while on a 30-minute phone call can gain as much as 1,800 steps.
- A 15-minute lunch break stroll may net 2,000 or more steps.
- Walking to a working colleague as compared to sending an email can earn about 60 steps.
- The 15 minutes after dinner stroll may net 1,700 to 2,000 steps.

LENGTH OF TIME PER DAY

One hour of walking is equivalent to about 15 minutes of running or any other high-impact exercise.

Walking briskly for about 90 minutes a day, 7 days a week burns, about 3,000 calories; a half-hour period is somewhat minimal and can account for about 1,500 calories.

Proper dieting plus 30 minutes vigorous walking each day for 5 days per week: anticipate a loss of about 2 lb (0.9 kg) per month. This adds up to 24 lb (11 kg approximately) per year.

It is to be noted that length of time walking per day can be done in one shift or in multiple time periods within the day. Whatever the pattern, the effectiveness achieved is the same.

COMPARATIVE BODY WEIGHT, WALKING PACE, AND CALORIE BURN

The term "moderate intensity" crops up quite frequently in this type of discussion on many aspects of physical activity. Keep in mind that the general definition for this term is equivalent to exceeding three times the energy consumption of rest.

It follows, therefore, that individual exertion at this intensity varies according to a person's fitness level. The result can vary between young and older adults. Consider moderate walking speed as 3.5 miles an hour, allowing for carrying on a conversation without noticeable pauses between words.

Walking at 2 miles per hour (a stroll) with a 150- to 155-lb body weight, one can anticipate a burn of 176 calories per hour, taking 20 hours to burn 1 lb. Walking at 3 miles an hour (4.8 kph)—that is, 4 kilometers per hour with 1mph equaling 1.61 kph; 1 lb = 0.45kg; 1 mile in 15 minutes equals 6.44 kph—approximates achieving 232 calories per hour. This means 15 hours to burn off 1 pound (0.45 kg). Increase the pace to 4 miles an hour (6.44 kph), the projection becomes 352 calories per hour and the burning of 1 pound is achieved in less than 10 hours.

Calorie-burn efficiency declines with an increase in body weight, all other things being equal.

It is suggested that 1 hour of moderate walking every day allows a person to lose their weight in calories; for example, if you weigh 160 lb, you can lose 160 calories. However, a moderately obese person doing moderate physical activity, such as brisk walking (or biking), may accomplish as much as a 350 calorie burn in 1 hour. In order to really challenge the cardiovascular system and achieve the increased demand on the heart, it is necessary to rev up the pace and intensity of the activity.

Some additional projected benefits:

- Walking briskly, 15 minutes a day, is associated with a lifespan gain of about 2 years; 1 hour a day, a 4-year gain in lifespan.
- Brisk walking 40 minutes a day, 4 days a week, can improve erectile function in men (Greger, 2019).

EXERCISE ACTIVITY REQUIRED TO BALANCE FOOD INTAKE

It takes about 3 miles of running on the same day to erase the potential fat deposit from eating two chicken legs boiled with skin removed; the food calorie effect being in excess of 300 calories and one mile of running burns 125 calories.

Similarly, consuming a super-sized fries or a choice of chicken salad over garden salad also means an extra 3 miles of walking/running on the same day. It takes a quarter mile of jogging to counter each bite on a Snickers bar or 1 hour of brisk walking to counter the calorie intake from a slice of pizza.

Most drinks, snacks, and processed junk food add calories at a rate of about 70 per minute; this means that it only takes about 5 minutes of snacking to wipe out a whole hour of exercise.

A serious lesson emerging from these projections which must guide the behaviour of an obese person is that you cannot party or attend a wedding feast, fish fry, or other cultural event with a focus on food consumption with lots of sugary beverages or a few bottles of beer. The resulting process of gobbling food way beyond reasonable satiation cannot be balanced by a plan to burn it off with a half-hour walk the next day. There is no evidence that provides the go ahead for such foolish, repetitive behaviour if you already have an obese problem.

Keep in mind what we may call the "Triple F" formula for walking exercise: the faster, further, and more frequently that you walk, the greater the benefits. Alternatively, increased calorie burn can also be achieved by increasing exercise intensity. Increase the pace by running instead of walking, or add intervals of more challenging terrain, hills, or stairs.

It is generally agreed that a regular and daily brisk walk can help strengthen bones and muscles; assist in the management of heart disease, high blood pressure, and type 2 diabetes; achieve mood improvement; improve balance and coordination; and, from the point of interest for obese persons, help to maintain a healthy weight including putting a dent in the visceral fat around the waist.

WALKING INCORPORATED WITH HIIT

The interval exercise pattern is already explained in Part 1 of this section. Interval walking is reported to lower blood sugar levels, regulate female hormones, and increase production of mood busting brain chemicals.

An interesting take off from interval training has been referred to as "wogging"; the application of walk/jog intervals—quite a boon to individuals who have limited time allotment for the struggle. Overall findings suggest some caution again in anticipation of total outcome from this strategy over a period of time. It would appear that there is moderate benefit in performance result from HIIT in terms of significant weight or body fat benefit as compared to standard engagement in continuous moderate intensity activity over a comparative period.

NORDIC POLE WALKING

I feel obliged to include a commentary on Nordic pole walking (NPW), also known as Nordic walking, which I have been practicing, even though with less sustainability than I would like. I do not hesitate to recommend this form of exercise to anyone, especially older adults.

NPW is an effective low-impact outdoor physical activity suitable for all ages and fitness levels; like skiing, it impacts all the major muscle groups in the body. It originated in Scandinavia and has become the fastest growing outdoor activity around the globe. In some countries, the cost of participation in organised programmes is paid by health insurance companies. About 5 years ago, it was estimated that over 15 million Europeans were engaged in Nordic pole walking.

The activity involves walking with a pair of poles used somewhat similar to the act of cross-country skiing. The proper use of light poles helps to keep the upper body in the fitness game, helps with stability, improves posture, and lessens the impact of walking on joints and muscles—in particular, hips, knees, and lower back.

The activity offers a range of flexibility in style, ranging from basic, relaxed walking with moderate pole pushing to a more aggressive arm swinging style using more powerful pole pushing (planting the pole vertically in the correct position at the side of the foot) with clear evidence of the muscular rhythm impacting, in particular, the upper body and facilitating an upright posture. Certified courses and instructors are widely available in many countries. [Schwanbeck, K [2018]

An important research finding is that NPW burns about 20% more calories over a 1-mile course compared to ordinary walking.

This form of exercise is increasingly being used by physiotherapists, is incorporated in rehabilitation programmes for a variety of conditions, and is finding favour in the early stages of Parkinson's disease. Most important is that the participants are almost oblivious of the extra burn with respect to levels of exertion felt during the exercise. It is said to give patients a good total body and cardiovascular workout without being exhausting.

Some summary pointers on the increased health benefits from scientific and clinical studies on NWP, as reported by Nordixx Pole Walking, Canada, are:

- Burns up to 46% more calories than ordinary walking.
- Increases heart and cardiovascular training by 25%
- Incorporates 90% of all body muscles in a single exercise and increases endurance of arm muscles and neck and shoulder muscles by 38%
- It takes only 30 minutes of NWP versus 55 minutes of regular walking to achieve the same training effects
- In people with type 2 diabetes, it improves diabetes metabolism, reduces insulin resistance, and reduces medication drastically within 3 months
- Reduces high blood pressure by 18 mmHg within 8 weeks
- Increases production of "positive" hormones
- Supports stress management and mental disorders
- Develops upright body posture

SUMMARY

Greger (2019) reports on the pooled results of 22 studies of walking for weight loss. It is an encouraging projection that that an average of 45 minutes or so of brisk walking, 4 times a week for 3–4 months, removes nearly 6 lb of body fat and also takes down that waist measurement by 1 inch.

Overall, the reported results for walking as a form of exercise may sound somewhat unencouraging for individuals looking for rapid success; however, it is necessary for the obese individual to understand that walking as the sole initiative for weight management is serious business. Considering that there are 3,500 calories in every pound of fat, at 100 calories per mile, this averages walking 35 miles to burn 3,500 calories. However, if 50% of calories burnt are derived almost equally from stored fat or carbohydrates, it really means walking 70 miles to lose a full pound of fat; a daunting task!

Remember: three extra miles to counteract the potential fat deposit from two chicken legs!

Here is some fundamental information relating to the structure of the human body and the special significance of walking. While there may be slight variation in numbers from different sources, it is quite clear that the muscle and bone structure of the lower body is critical information demanding special attention with respect to general health and management of the ageing process. Indications are that there are about 207 bones in the human adult body with about one quarter of them in the foot and ankle, containing some 26 bones, 30 to 33 joints, and over 100 muscles, tendons, and ligaments. Both feet account for 52 bones. This overall structure provides for core management of support, balance, and mobility.

Finally, if it is true that ageing starts "from the feet up"; the significance of walking and other related exercises signals importance in an exercise regime for all ages. Consider the saying that "exercising the feet is a life-long task."

Information on designing exercise programmes for walking is available on the internet; additional suggested walking routines are provided in a few publications. Simplification of explanation can go a long way in the search.

Here is an abbreviated listing of tips to consider in planning for and executing workout and circuit programmes for walking aimed at achieving good health in a general sense and more so if the intention is to achieve successful weight management.

- Good posture and purposeful movement; i.e., shoulders pulled back and keeping the spine tall or straight.
- Train the abs, such as tucking in the belly button towards the spine. The aim is to engage that deep muscle running across the lower abdominal region.
- Plan your routine and get good gear: sturdy walking shoes, suitable clothing for prevailing weather, lightweight water bottle, a pedometer and/or heart rate monitor.

- Select the travel course: road condition, lighting for late evening walks, safe neighbourhoods, convenient public parks.
- Remember to stretch. It helps to avoid painful discomfort in between or on the following days.
- Warming up for an exercise regime is always emphasised; remember also to cool down.
- Tracking your progress can assist in monitoring effective execution and adjustment where necessary. Use your pedometer or fitness tracker (calculate steps, distance). Possibly daily weighing if fat loss is an important goal.
- Exercise with committed company. This helps with keeping up the motivation level, enjoying the activity, changing routines, and interpersonal accountability.
- Listening to music is said to increase performance and reduce tension in the passing of time (Dr. Oz, 2020).

Walking is reported as having a host of benefits: a remarkable reduction in risk of breast cancer, type 2 diabetes, depression, anxiety, insomnia, and stress. It facilitates weight loss, reduction of blood pressure, and boosts brain health.

It contributes to the building of muscles which provide support to bones, ligaments, and tendons. Moderate intensity walking can supposedly prevent weight gain in as little as 150 minutes per week; within the sports world, the recommendation increases to 250 minutes. There is also a reported indication, based upon analysis of some 800 research studies, that 1 in 7 cases of Alzheimer disease could be prevented if individuals simply followed the recommendation to walk briskly for 30 minutes at least 5 times a week.. Physical activity reduced by 40% the likelihood of developing the disease.

Inter alia, walking has been referred to, in wholesome and humorous terms, as "an organic, natural, gluten-free, fat free, toxin-free, meditative experience" (Teychenne and Miller, 2020).Keep in mind also that walking has the lowest quit rate of any type of exercise.

CHAPTER 11
INDIVIDUAL AND SOCIETAL COSTS: THE PREVALENCE OF OVERWEIGHT AND OBESITY ISSUES

THE INDIVIDUAL

Losing weight is challenging but all indications are that early intervention makes it easier to turn around the potential problems. Where possible, a parent assisting a child to manage their weight management while young, or even in the teen years, is an advantage. Overweight teens tend to become overweight adults who may well develop long-term medical problems, such as diabetes and a range of other health problems.

We must also take heed that overweight teenagers are likely to experience teasing and being bullied at school, humiliated, and also being ostracized. They may, themselves, develop a tendency to engage in bullying behaviour. Personal seclusion is a possibility. All this may be associated with mental health problems such as depression.

Both youth and adults can experience the creation of negative self-images, feelings of demotivation, and a definite lack of self-confidence.

The effects on the social and sexual life of the obese individual can become very evident. The associated hormonal imbalance and lower testosterone levels can literally prevent or at least diminish capacity for sexual intimacy, definitely affecting, possibly ruining, both aspects of the adult life. Testosterone is the primary male sex hormone in males. It plays a key role in humans with respect to the development of male reproductive tissues such as the testes and prostate. It is also significant in the promotion of secondary sexual characteristics. In particular, reduced levels may lead to both erectile dysfunction and increased inhibition of sexual desire in men.

The best response can be very complicated. I begin by sharing the following quotation (Greger, 2019):

> The largest study in history on the health effects of being overweight analyzed data from more than fifty million people in nearly two hundred countries and found that too much excess body weight accounts for the premature deaths of about four million people every year. Most of these deaths are from heart disease, but the researchers found "convincing" or "probable" evidence linking obesity to twenty different disorders.

The World Health Organization (WHO) classifies obesity as one of the most significant health risks in modern society. Looking closely at the health issues of the obese individual, numerous areas of concern emerge. Greger (2019) makes reference to a veritable alphabet soup of these potential health concerns. A brief, selected listing illustrates the enormity of the situation.

Arthritis. Arthritis is the most common joint disease in the world. It can worsen to become rheumatoid arthritis and increase the risk of gout, another inflammatory joint disease. Weight reduction may minimise the need for knee replacement surgery. It is noted that losing 20 pounds of fat might be regarded as an alternative to knee replacement surgery, especially considering that nearly one in two hundred knee replacement patients die within 90 days of surgery.

Back Pain. Being overweight increases the risk of lower back pain, disc degeneration, and other related conditions. Clogged lumbar arteries that feed the spine can lead to deprivation of oxygen and nutrients to related areas.

Blood Pressure. Excess visceral fat can compress the kidneys, squeeze sodium back into the blood stream, and increase blood pressure. Disastrous health implications arise from combined high blood pressure and obesity. Indications are that a 9-pound loss in body weight can lower blood pressure in a manner equivalent to the effect of about a 50% reduction in salt.

Cancer and the Immune System. There is a definite link between obesity and cancer. Excess body fat raises the risk of most cancers. Post-menopausal, obese women have increased levels of estrogen circulating in their bloodstream, with the increased risk of developing and dying from breast cancer.

In relation to cancer, natural killer cells are the first line of defense of our immune system; their function is severely impaired by obesity.

Diabetes. Obesity is considered the single most important risk factor for the development of type 2 diabetes, which is now considered to be the leading cause of kidney failure, lower limb amputations, and adult-onset blindness.

Encephalopathy. "Encephalopathy" means a group of conditions which cause brain disease or dysfunction., appearing, inter alia, as confusion, memory loss, or personality changes. It can be life threatening, even leading to permanent brain damage or coma when severe. [https://Cleveland clinic.org>health]

There is strong indication of significantly increased chances of cognitive decline, loss of brain tissue, and various other brain conditions, including depression. Dementia and Alzheimer's are indicated, with a one-third higher risk for overweight individuals and a 90% greater risk for midlife obesity with respect to the onset of dementia.

Fertility. Issues related to pregnancy and impaired infertility are indicated for both men and women. The presence of excess fat is of concern in relation to critical male and female hormones, testosterone and estrogen respectively.

A shift from "obese" to "just overweight" is reported to potentially raise testosterone levels in the blood of men by 13%. Obese women of child-bearing age are more likely to experience difficulty in conceiving. Also, obesity during pregnancy means a greater likelihood of complications both during and after pregnancy.

Excess fat in the pubic area of men and the condition referred to as "buried", "trapped," "concealed," or "inconspicuous" penis is a matter of interest; that is, issues of inflammation and surgical intervention related to "Free Willy"!

Gallstones. Gallbladder issues relate to the number one digestive reason people are hospitalised, supposedly, in the developed world; 80%–90% of gallstones are made of crystalised cholesterol in the gall bladder. The most common cause and effect factor may well be obesity, increasing the risk of the condition as much as sevenfold.

Heart Disease. Excess body weight, regardless of the cause, is related to deaths from cardiovascular disease.

Jaundice. Besides the easily seen locations of fat accumulation, such as our thighs, bellies, and perhaps bottoms, excess fat enters some of our internal organs. A large percentage of individuals (even exceeding 90%) with severe obesity may have fatty infiltration of the liver. This can lead to inflammation, cirrhosis, and liver cancer.

Kidneys. Obesity is one of the strongest risk factors for serious kidney disease problems. Excess body weight means increased demand on metabolic function of the organ. The increased pressure can lead to damaged organs and an increased risk of kidney failure.

How Important is the Genetic Factor?

While it is an encouraging mantra to take note of the saying that one's DNA does not inevitably determine the level of obesity which prevails in a life long context, it is important to pay attention to the cumulative scientific conclusions on this matter. The individual needs to know the full struggle to be faced in the battle of the bulge. One Canadian website [https://obesitycanada.ca/understanding obesity] gives great emphasis to the DNA factor. Obesity is referred to as a brain related disorder, the hypothalmus playing an important role in the hunger-satiety continuum. The simple and clear statement is:

Obesity is increasingly being touted as highly genetic; as such, this means that the more of those genes you have, the more probable it is that you will develop obesity by age 18.

Severe obesity will more likely be expressed with greater numbers, genes dictating as much as much as 70 to 80 % of our BMI discussed earlier. Mothers who are obese at conception or gain significant weight during the pregnancy are more likely to give birth to large babies. We take note that Greger [2019] writes that the genetic contribution at the time " may be small".

Modern-Day, Costly Treatments for Stubborn Obesity Problems

Increasingly, when individuals have tried lengthy pursuits of varying endless exercise routines, numerous diets and pills, and a range of weight loss plans, they may decide on treatment by surgery (bariatic surgery) and associated techniques.

Liposuction. Liposuction is reportedly the most popular cosmetic surgery globally, with as much as 20 pounds of fat being sucked out from total body fat. Reportedly, even a 5%–10% reduction of body weight in fat can lead to meaningful improvements in health: blood pressure, blood sugars, inflammation, cholesterol, and triglycerides. This is not necessarily the result of massive liposuction invasions. Caution is suggested with respect to expectations, since the real problems related to excess fat may be limited in relation to subcutaneous fat compared to the dangerous visceral fat surrounding and infiltrating the inner organs.

Liposculpting. Different from liposuction, liposculpting is also referred to as transdermal technology, the targeted areas being stomach, legs, arms, chin, butt, and face. There is a focus on herbal and homeopathic remedies and can be executed without patients leaving their homes.

Stomach Stapling and Sleeve Gastrectomy (Sleeve Weight Surgery). These are varying surgical modifications aimed at reducing the active stomach surface. They may involve an internal bypass procedure, such as bypassing much of the small intestine, a kind of rearranging of the anatomy. They can also involve a carving out or complete removal of about as much as 20 feet of small intestine, leaving a small bit of stomach and limiting food intake as a result of substantial reduction in appetite and cravings. Results may lead to more than 50% loss of excess weight.

Indications are a greater likelihood of numerous complications being encountered including osteoporosis, vitamin and nutrient deficiencies, post-operational eating behaviours, even brain damage. Issues involving a return to the operating room, subsequent complications, and even death can be a cause for concern. Bariatric surgery has been reported to result in 55% to 75% of obese and super-obese diabetics attaining normal blood sugar levels quite soon after the procedure.

These procedures can be costly involving thousands of dollars. Low-cost offers (compared to North American costs) are offered in some countries with varying levels of success.

Clearly, individuals contemplating any form of bariatric surgery as an option in weight control ought to become well-informed about the advantages and disadvantages of the various procedures. It has been emphasised that bariatric surgery is not a quick fix. It is only the first step in decision to pursue a lifelong commitment to a healthy lifestyle. Thereafter, issues of diet, food intake, and exercise become crucial for sustained success. New behaviours become critical.

Emotional issues may well emerge and the understanding of the relationship between mental illness and obesity are important in a treatment regime. It is suggested that individuals undergoing bariatric surgery should undergo pre-surgical mental health screening by the appropriate medical personnel. Poor weight-loss outcome can lead to the emergence of significant risk factors, including mental health deterioration and depression. Suicidal issues and psychiatric stability are to be monitored.

Cryolipolysis (Cell Death). CoolSculpting is based upon the fact that fat cells in the body are more susceptible to cold injury compared to surrounding water-rich tissue in skin muscle. Controlled exposure to cold temperatures results in reduced subcutaneous fat at treatment site; the fat cells are frozen and permanently destroyed and finally removed by natural elimination, within a period of 2 to 6 months. Fat reduction by as much as 25% is indicated.

There is also a type of sculp surgery, which uses heat to target fat cells, again, leading to natural elimination.

The treatment is not advertised, so much with a focus on weight changes but more so as a way of achieving a redistribution of fat cells and a means of eliminating fat pockets, which have proven resistant to the normal procedures of diet and exercise. Focussed treatment areas include the abdomen, hips, bra-fat, inner and outer thighs, and chin. A full body exposure procedure is referred to as cryotherapy.

BROADER SOCIETAL COSTS

It is to be noted that on-the-job brazen discrimination and even a noticeable wage gap are real possibilities in the world of employment. There is a stigma associated with obesity. Even in small amounts, an obese condition is also known to affect the most intimate relationships; in a more general sense, low and negative self-esteem effects influence activity level and lifestyle, all of which are regarded with a capacity to stress partnerships, marriage, and other related intimate bonds.

Obese individuals are expected to die sooner. Being overweight, or any level of obesity, projects an earlier-than-normal demise from planet Earth. The evidence suggests that an approximate 12 pounds loss from just diet and exercise projects a 12% reduction in early mortality. The average age of death for an obese American is about 56 years, a massive reduction in life span (Bonham, 2020).

Individuals suffer mentally from the obesity condition through a host of circumstances. One Timothy reported a prolonged dietary descent as result of being raped at age 6; thereafter, for most of his life, food became his comfort and he was at war with his "overshadowing figure," married three times, "fighting for life, love and against loneliness." At age 50, he weighs over 500 pounds (Ramdeo, 2023).

Childhood obesity is now recognised as part of the global health crisis. While initially it was regarded as a problem in countries at the stage of economic transition, between developing and developed, some researchers conclude that the problem is at alarming levels in both developed and developing countries, and within all socio-economic groups and irrespective of age, sex or ethnicity. There is some variation in reporting with respect to age, socio economic status [SES] and gender within the country level of development. It is noted hat the prevalence of obesity may well be higher in western and industrialized countries

Childhood obesity is also associated with health conditions which can be costly to the national economy, Typical psychological conditions include anxiety, depression and low self esteem, Additional societal problems reported are bullying, the stigma of being obese and a reported lower quality of life . [Kosti, R.I., 2006 and Wang, Youfa et al., 2012] .

Studies have linked childhood obesity to a reduced attention span and impaired concentration and focus, serious issues related to career success in almost any area of choice (Melone, 2019).

An aversion to treating obese patients by medical staff is indicated.. They have been referred to as "awkward, unattractive, ugly, and noncompliant"; nurses have indicated being repulsed. Doctors turn away heavier, obese women, some setting definite weight limits for patience acceptance. Others, reportedly give less quality time to such patients and tend to build less emotional rapport, such that the authenticity of patient-physician relationship has been questioned (Greger, 2019).

Globally, obesity affects both developed and developing countries, impacting all age groups and socio-economic levels. Increases in the prevalence of obesity are more dramatic in societies in transition, that is, with an expanding middle class and particularly among the more affluent sections of those countries.

And there are suggestions from different quarters for direct government intervention in patterns of food consumption. It is noted, for example that Britons spend 3.9 billion pounds per year **on** confectionery compared to 2.2 billion pounds on fruits and vegetables [www.the guardian.com/society/2023/dec/04/cost-of-people-being-overweight].The food environment is considered to have moved beyond recognition into what is labeled as "obesogenic."

Projected data regarding numbers of individuals who are overweight in 2020 compared to 2035 indicates % for men and 18% for women in 2020 will rise to 23% for men and 27 % for women in 2035.; more than half the world's population in that age category will be obese,

According to English (2011), in the US, four out of five African American women, compared to about one half of white women, were obese or overweight in 2011. The National Centre for Health Statistics Centre for Disease Prevention and Control reports 49.6% prevalence for obesity among non-Hispanic black adults, 44.8% for Hispanic adults, 42.2% for non-Hispanic whites, and a much lower 17.4% for non-Hispanic Asian adults. For comparison by age, the prevalence figures were 40% for adults less than 40 years old, 44.8% for the 40 to 59 age group, and 42.8% for the group 60 years and over.

Data analysis indicated lower prevalence levels associated with higher education among both men and women with insignificant readings between non-Hispanic groups. Making comparisons on the basis of educational level and income proved to be more complex with differences by sex, race, and ethnicity. The continued worsening situation for the adult population is indicated by obesity prevalence rates for adults of 42.4% for 2017–2018, increasing more than 10% in less than 2 decades. The prevalence of adult severe obesity almost doubled within the same period, increasing from 4.7% to 9.2%. Research data also points to some significant differences between ethnic groupings and also on the basis of comparative social status.

For the USA, evidence suggests that an obese individual can incur very high extra costs in medical expenditure compared to an individual with a healthy weight. Obesity with its potential multiple complications can cost a company as much as US$10,000 per individual—much more in health coverage compared to leaner employees. Additional issues relating to an individual company may include absenteeism and a loss of productivity, disability pensions, and premature deaths. Many insurance companies, especially with respect to life insurance, charge higher premiums with increasing degrees of overweight. Projected costs over a lifetime have been estimated as high as US$200,000 for a single individual and about US$150 billion at the national level in the US.

Canadian statistical data indicate 63 %of Canadian adults as being obese or overweight in 2018 compared to 61.9% in 2015. Categorised obesity relate to about 29% of the adult population for 2021 but categorised overweight is indicated as much as 36% in 2022. Obesity prevalence is reportedly rising faster in rural areas (31.4 % in 2020) versus 25.6% in urban areas. Also, adult obesity is more prevalent among disadvantaged population groups, those who are underemployed or with lower education levels and lower incomes. [https://obesitycanada.ca/understanding-obesity/]

Research data (*Canadian Risk Factor Atlas,* 2020) has demonstrated a definite relationship between asthma and high BMI. Both Canada and the

US are reporting a rise in the incidence of asthma: dramatic increases in prevalence among children aged 0–14 for Canada and rising from 2.5% in 1979 to 11.2 % in 1995 over a period of 18 years. It is referred to as: "the most chronic disease among children and the leading cause for both school absenteeism and hospitalization" (Miller, 2022).

There is serious concern on the matter of obesity at the national level in the UK , considered to be "the most obese nation in Western Europe" Two thirds of adults are classed as overweight or obese and more than one-third of all children are considered obese. It is stated that obesity now causes more cancer than smoking.. Overall costs have soared from £58 billion in 2020 to almost £100 billion in 2023, taking into account the value of health lost through illness and disease; a situation considered to be" an absolute public health disaster" Similarly, the cost to people affected rose from 45.2 billion pounds to 63.1 billion pounds"[https:// The Guardian.com:society.UK.2023"]

The obesity issue is especially very serious in Latin America and the Caribbean. In a little over 4 decades ending in 2018, the prevalence of obesity among adults tripled to an average of one in four adults (25%), almost double the global average of 13.2%.

The situation is even worse in the Caribbean sub-region with over-weight, including obesity, ranging from a low of about 18.9% among some of the islands to as high as 31.6% in the Bahamas and an even higher figure for Jamaica, 54%. That means one in every two persons and the reality being that two thirds of Jamaican women 15 years or older were over-weight or obese in 2018.

In the Cayman Islands, 70% of men and women are considered over-weight and more than 30% as obese. The rate of obesity in women is about 10% higher than among men (Bonham, 2020).

In Barbados, it is estimated that one in three children are "over-nour-ished" (overweight or obese); the situation being linked to a dietary pattern high in salt, sugar, and fat (lots of junk food) together with established patterns of imbibing sugary, carbonated drinks.

It may be somewhat amusing to note that Nauru, the smallest island nation in the world, is rated as the most obese country globally with an obesity rate of 61% in early 2023, supposedly due to the shift from traditional diet to Western-style diet combined with an increasingly sedentary lifestyle.

Against all this background information, it is clear that obesity is recognised as a serious global health issue. National governance in some countries are commencing serious policy interventions especially as they apply to food consumption. An important Canadian statistic which fires the need for continuing research is that most studies indicate that achieved weight loss resulting from dietary and exercise interventions "disappear" within 4 to 7 years. . [https://obesitycanada,ca/understanding -obesity/]

SUMMARY

At this point, we are at the end of the informational initiative of this comprehensive review on obesity. The how, why, which, where, and when of overweight and obesity issues have been extensively reviewed, at times with personal commentaries. This chapter moves the dialogue beyond the details of related science and folklore as it affects the individual on to the global overview. It is an increasingly important subject area without geographical boundaries.

This review of information on issues related obesity ought to be sufficiently convincing for the average reader that acknowledgement of retained excess body fat combined with a full awareness of the potential consequences should serve as a call to action for any individual faced with an obesity problem.

The fact is that being overweight carries a reservoir of potential risks that can significantly shorten the life span or facilitate a life of severe health challenges for the average individual. A very wide range of health issues may emerge from any combination of having a sustained obese condition and the adoption of an associated unhealthy lifestyle.

If you conclude that you have an excessive weight or obesity problem, try to minimise your susceptibility to a host of potential health issues. I urge the reader to give thought to one of them in particular: metabolic syndrome and its relationship with leaky gut, covered in great detail in an earlier chapter.

The reader is provided with a peek into national and international significance and a clear indication that the real cost of obesity is a matter which demands attention within the scope of personal, national, and regional concern.

CHAPTER 12
SELECTED TIPS: MANAGING LIFESTYLE CHANGES CONSIDERED NECESSARY FOR COMBATING OBESITY

THIS FINAL CHAPTER represents an attempt at a focussed summary of key pointers, provided for routine review by the individual who faces up to the task of managing an overweight and most likely obese condition, all in the pursuit of a healthy and happier life. This chapter is a simplified encapsulation, under 17 subheads, of selected important information discussed in previous chapters.

The presentation facilitates a periodic and quick review, when necessary, of salient points intended to keep the reader on track with respect to guidance for day-to-day decisions related to the necessary changes in lifestyle, such as are most likely to succeed in the context of combating obesity.

A weekly review of the content is recommended for the first 6 months of a planned effort to tackle the issue of personal obesity.

Overall, there is no magic formula of any type, no single variable that will lead to sustained success in battling obesity.

THE PSYCHOLOGY OF SELF DETERMINATION AND SELF-MANAGEMENT

Understand and accept the significant advantages in adopting an approach which necessitates behaviours which help to self-check and manage progress on a regular basis.

You may need to accept a kind of draconian discipline to be successful at achieving that change in lifestyle, which is necessary in your quest to manage obesity. It may well be a "total makeover," resulting in the abandonment of long-standing old habits.

In determining the totality of what is necessary, understand and accept that there is no shortcut; do not waste time searching for a single pill, lotion, potion, concoction, or esoteric diet. There is no single magic formula that fits all.

WHAT AND HOW MUCH YOU EAT

The Calorie Dense versus Dilute Approach

Understand and embrace the significance of "calorie dense" as compared to "calorie dilute" in choosing what foods and drinks you intake daily. This necessitates a new awareness and alertness of the calorie density of just about everything you eat; this is different compared to attempting to count the calories you consume, a much more demanding routine. This new awareness can provide considerable, beneficial guidance in managing daily eating patterns or habits.

The basic principle is to select food items which are non-starchy and are clearly calorie dilute and water-dense or high in water content. They offer the advantage of almost empty calories. Celery, cucumber, turnips, cauliflower, squash, bean sprouts, zucchini, and kale are essentially water trapped in vegetable form.

In the same context, minimise the intake of calorie-dense food types. A good idea will be to eat a salad at least once a day, such as at lunch. Take note that vegetable oils, including the popular olive oil, are calorie dense. One extra tablespoon of olive oil on your salad adds 120 calories. Nuts, like oils, contain lots of fat and are calorie dense; not much more than an ounce (a handful) is recommended daily.

The Calorie Intake Count (the Burn) Approach

This approach necessitates building knowledge of the actual calorie content of the food you consume; for example, consuming a candy bar means approximately 150 calories, equivalent to about 30 cups of lettuce. A single meal at a fast-food restaurant, especially with adolescents, can mean an intake in excess of 1,600 calories.

It is necessary to create a calorie deficit (burn more calories than are consumed). A focus on fruit and vegetables facilities the lower calorie intake, while simultaneously ensuring a level of fibre content which promotes a satiated feeling. When we consume more calories (energy) than is used up in the numerous metabolic processes, which take place within our bodies, the excess is stored in different locations as body fat.

If you consistently burn all the calories you consume in the course of a day, your weight is maintained. Consume more energy (calories) than you expend, and your weight will increase. Keep in mind that a few dozen calories on each and every occasion, taking place sufficiently frequently, adds up and can defeat the ultimate objective in the control of obesity.

Remember: burn it or churn it.

There is an alternative point of view: do not focus on the numbers but take note of "how you feel" after a meal. However, this is a package deal to which due attention must be given to understanding blood sugar, the microbiome, and a host of other factors affecting obesity.

The temptation of second helpings must be resisted.

From the calorie point of view, achieving successful weight loss points to approximate daily consumption of a maximum of 1,200 calories for women and 1,500 for men.

Soup lovers have slimmer waists and lower body weight; soup as a first course usually leads to smaller amounts consumed of a main course.

CARBOHYDRATES, PROTEINS, AND FATS

As a general principle, reduce carbohydrates and consume more protein. Eating protein burns more calories at rest.

Fats

Keep a close look at your source of fats. Know the sources of good fats as compared to bad fats.

Saturated fats contain a high proportion of fatty acid molecules and are less healthy for dietary intake. They should not exceed 10% of your daily intake of calories and sources to watch include animal products (cheese, butter).

Unsaturated fats, in general, provide a healthy group of fats. Good sources are fish (salmon), vegetable oils (soya bean, canola, olive), walnuts, and avocados. Source your fat mostly from lean meats, fish, and heart healthy oils.

Trans-fats are to be avoided; like saturated fats, they carry an indication of high cholesterol and increased risk of heart disease. They are found naturally in meat (all kinds) and dairy. They are a form of unsaturated fat. Common sources include deep-fried foods, ready-to-eat frozen foods, commercially baked goods, and sweet and salty snacks foods of all kinds, including cakes and cookies. The general principle is to avoid processed foods as much as possible.

Reduce red meat and replace with lean meat, such as chicken and fish. Replace a meal of meat and vegetables with fruit, vegetables, whole grains, and beans. Mushrooms are good replacement for meat. They represent approximately 100 calories per pound and can reduce calorie intake by 50%.

FIBRE CONTENT

A plant-based diet has clear advantages in reducing calorie consumption. It tends to be very satisfying and a significant number of calories remain trapped (encapsulated).

It helps fill you up, eat right, and still lose weight. High-fibre content goes a long way in providing a feeling of satiation, when eating, thereby affecting the quantity of food consumed at any one time Eat the skin of apples and pears..

Highly processed foods and most leafy veggies are most likely void of significant fibre and nutrient content.

Good fibre content affects the quality of bacteria in the microbiome; fibre-eating bacteria are important for the quality of gut health.

Consumption of a plant-based diet provide numerous advantages in the control of obesity; fibre content affects the rate of digestion and the rate of sugar absorption—that is, the important matters of blood sugar level control, fat absorption, fat deposit, and so forth.

WHEN WE EAT (TIMING)

In a general sense, time of day when critical meals are consumed is important. Our circadian rhythm or body clock comes into play; the cycle varying with temperature and light. It affects every tissue and organ in the body. Food eaten too late in the evening or at night tends to leave more fat behind when compared to the same intake during the normal waking day.

The Night Fast: Restricting Food Consumption

The core aim here is to restrict eating to achieve a long fasting period between further intake, be it hours or days. For individuals who are constant nibblers once they are awake, this is a tough challenge. The reasoning weighs in on capturing the benefits of the circadian rhythm to which the body is subjected.

Controlling evening food consumption in the last meal of the day is critical. Recommendations vary for taking the last meal, such as 6 p.m. or 7 p.m. The general objective is to attain a long period of fasting between the last meal and the first the next morning, usually 12 hours if possible. The fewer calories after sundown, the more likely for success in the battle of the bulge.

Do not eat meals, in general, while distracted, such as looking at TV or when actively engaged in phone calls. (See also notes regarding the timing of eating in relation to exercise schedule.)

Eating Breakfast

There are positive indications of clear advantages in maintaining the breakfast habit, usually within 1–2 hours of waking up.

FRONT-LOADING YOUR CALORIES

There is an advantage to consuming most of your calories early in the day when hunger hormones are less active. Consuming larger amounts of calories at breakfast can double the amount of weight loss and reduce waistline girth compared to consumption at dinner time. Remember: *Breakfast like a king, lunch like a prince, and dinner like a pauper.* A variant of this is: *Eat breakfast yourself, share lunch with a friend, give dinner away to your enemy.*

Whole fruit is often a popular part of the breakfast menu, especially given its association with fibre; however, the presence of large amounts of sugar (fructose) can have negative effects. Leave it out if your obesity problem is a serious challenge. Aim for fruits with a low glycemic index, such as apples, grapefruit, and berries.

Beware of bread, *especially white bread*, and the wheat belly condition. Bread, by any name, is best left out of the shopping cart if beating the battle of the bulge is a serious undertaking.

HOW YOU CONSUME

Chewing Your Food = More Time in the Mouth

It is advantageous to practice thorough chewing of food; food intake can be reduced by as much as one third. Slower eating leads to a feeling of increased satiation and lower food consumption.

Slow down your eating; give the brain time to inform the stomach of a sufficiency of intake and to process the meal. There is an old formula: one chew for each tooth (chew each mouthful 32 times). Overweight and obese persons tend to chew each mouthful significantly less than individuals with more normal weight levels. Eat until you are satisfied, avoid getting to the point of feeling full.

It is possible to facilitate longer time periods in the mouth by taking smaller bites, eating slower, or chewing longer. However, if it is achieved by increasing the time in the mouth, it can lead to lower caloric intake.

SNACKING: SOME RECOMMENDED OPTIONS

Snacking takes place quite frequently and is often focussed on the wrong foods; the result is a pile-up of lots of calories and pounds of fat than is expected.

Food snacking, typically composed of drinks, processed foods, baked goods, generally indicates an intake of about 70 calories per minute. This means that snacking can easily neutralise the intended effects of an exercise programme. In essence, 5 minutes of snacking can wipe out an hour of exercise. If you must snack, choose snack items that will minimise the elevation of your insulin levels. Eat with awareness, maintain consciousness of your eating. Do not accommodate picking non stop behaviour.

Recommended snack items include: a handful of nuts, a piece of fruit, baby carrots, berries or grapes, apples and peanut butter, cucumber slices in a salsa sauce, celery sticks dipped in ranch dressing, steamed broccoli, soya sauce on steamed cabbage.

EXERCISE

The overwhelming point of view is that incorporation of some measure of meaningful physical is necessary. Keep the three essentials in mind: what goes in, what comes out, and the need to move the body to accomplish the expenditure (burn) of energy. Burning off calories is hard work.

Walking: Time, Speed, and Calorie (Energy) Burn

Here are some selected examples to guide your estimation of what is required to meet appropriate goals.

1. **Strolling:** walking leisurely i.e. 2 miles per hour (30 minutes per mile). With a bodyweight of 150/155 lb = 176 calories burn per hour (20 hours to burn 1 lb)
2. **Striding:** 3 mph = 20 minutes per mile; 3 miles per hour approximates a burn of 232 calories per hour = 15 hrs to burn 1 pound.
3. **Brisk walking:** about 3.5 miles (6.4 km) an hour; 17 minutes per mile. To achieve a 15-minute-mile walking pace, necessary to walk at 4–5 miles (6–8 km per hour) i.e. you can talk but cannot sing a song.
    a. 30 minutes approximates 150 calories burned
    b. 90 minutes per day x 7 days per week = 3,000 calories
    c. 45 minutes per day x 7 days per week = 1,500 calories

If you were to run a mile, you'd burn approximately 125 calories.

Volume is important; At least 300 minutes of exercise a week seem to be necessary to achieve any significant weight loss (Greger, 2019).

Remember, you can split up the targeted programme within a single day; if necessary, sneak in separate bits and cumulate to the targeted amount to be achieved.

The Importance of Matching Energy Burn with Food Consumption

Beware of the tendency towards a rise in intake as calorie expenditure increases through exercise. Be aware of the real demands on physical exercise to neutralize excessive calorie intake.

Two boiled chicken legs with skin removed: (approximately 350 calories) equals 3 miles of running.

One slice of pizza (300 calories) is one-hour brisk walking. Avoid the willpower booby trap: sweat in the gym for 1 hour, burn 300 calories, and follow this up by consuming 500 calories—a meat sausage with fries!

Timing of Exercise: When to Exercise

Timing is important in facilitating maximum burn with an exercise regime.

Muscular activity after eating reduces blood spikes and diverts blood flow away from the intestines with a result of slower glucose absorption into the blood stream, since some of it is directed to use by working muscles rather than accumulation for storage. Exercising for 10–15 minutes makes a meaningful difference in the management of blood sugar spikes.

In general, it is advantageous to exercise in a fasted (before food) condition; a general recommendation is 6 hours after the previous meal and before the next meal, especially before any breakfast, lunch, or dinner. Pre-meal activity heralds significant differences in achieving fat burn.

The recommendation is different for diabetics, who must adhere to appropriate advice; exercise post-dinner, or whichever is the largest meal, becomes especially important.

Facilitating Maintenance of Exercise Schedules

Beware of the temptation to treat yourself to excessive calorie intake post-exercise activity. Think of ways to make exercise enjoyable, such as walking with friends or listening to music.

The "buddy system"—exercising with companions—also facilitates sustainability of the proposed exercise programme; one of the best ways to cement an exercise habit. Friends keep us accountable (not letting down each other) and relieve boredom. This can take about 6 weeks.

Without the buddy approach, one may constantly be looking for the right time which may never come! Mini workouts (separate periods in one day) can help, such as a jog in the morning, a walk at lunch, a few crunches, or a 10- to 15-minute walk before bed.

Stretching

Stretching is an important part of a good exercise session. Varying recommendations emphasise pre and post physical exercise. Indications are that there are advantages for both warming up and cooling down in the exercise programme.

DNA AND BODY-FAT ACCUMULATION: KEEP HOPE ALIVE

Individuals and their eating habits vary in the extent to which they accumulate excess fat and gain weight. Be attuned to your personal situation, issues of inheritance (genes), and environment. *Understand, however, that in most cases DNA inheritance does not confine any individual to a* lifetime of inevitable obesity.

Your DNA inheritance does not seal your fate at birth; your genes are not your destiny.

FOOD ADDITIVES: SPICES, HERBS, AND BERRIES

Spices and Herbs.
The following spices and herbs are all considered useful and effective in weight control. They .are likely to have a major effect with regard to appetite suppression and may also help to rev up metabolic rate and increase fat burn.
- Cumin: effective and low-cost; add ½ teaspoon lunch or dinner.
- Turmeric: suggested as being effective in facilitating weight control.

- Garlic: a ¼ teaspoon of garlic powder daily is a low-cost reducer of body fat.
- Ginger: ¼ to 1½ teaspoons per day
- Green Tea extract appears to have positive effect.

Pepper and Peppery Condiments

A range of pepper sources can contribute in varying degrees to weight loss when added to the daily diet. They include raw, whole pepper (jalapeno, bell), pepper powders, or flakes (½ a teaspoon).

My personal experience is that adding pepper or peppery preparations to salads and soups contributes to the overall taste. This may not be welcomed by persons who do not like or use pepper routinely.

Fruit and Berries

See notes under "Fruit at Breakfast Time."

A wide variety of fruits are recommended for regular consumption; these include citrus fruit, pineapple, and berries (blueberries, raspberries, and blackberries).

WATER

There is a miracle to the role of water in achieving good health in general. Water is critical in the struggle against overweight and obesity. Remember that adequate hydration is of significance in every possible cellular process in the human body; it affects the metabolic rate [number of calories used] in bodily chemical reactions and is significant in achieving and maintaining weight loss.

Drinking water before each meal (pre-eating water consumption) is a general recommendation and can facilitate reduced calorie consumption.

Late-night snacking is a serious hindrance to effective weight control. A glass of water can reduce the tendency towards late-night snacking. Do not mistake thirst for hunger; very often, a glass of water is much healthier than reaching for snack food and reduces the intake of unwanted calories.

Avoid purchase of and keep out of sight sugary drinks and diet sodas. Their substitution with pure water, on a regular basis, can reduce calorie intake by 235 calories per day; at times, a reduction as high as 400%.

A glass of safe tap water four times a day has the potential to burn an extra 100 calories. As a general rule, aim at consuming 6–8 glasses of water daily.

Always remember the importance of water content in food choices. In this regard, remember the significance of pre- or front-loading a meal with low-calorie-dense foods, which give a feeling of satisfaction or fullness; for example, 1 cup of celery equals only 16 calories. Vegetables with both high-water and fibre content can make a difference; develop the habit of using salads extensively. It is more effective to preload with low-calorie-dense salads compared to consuming them alongside the meal. Good choices include celery, cucumbers, zucchini, tomatoes, lettuce, and kale.

At the same time, beware of fatty salad dressings; some of them can quadruple the calorie intake. A salad is only as good as the dressing used. Some useful measurements:

1 tbsp = 16 g

1 cup = 250 g

100 g of Wish Bone Blue Cheese Dressing = 450 calories

100 g of vinaigrette = 449 calories

Keep in mind that, generally speaking, vinaigrettes tend to be the healthier dressings as they are usually balsamic or oil and vinegar. Some vinaigrettes are as low as 50–70 calories. Anything reading "creamy," such as ranch or Caesar dressings, are less healthy.

As noted elsewhere, increasing water intake is an important aspect of effective poo management. Water lubricates the alimentary canal and facilitates movement; very often when the exit movement from the gut seems impossible, experience the successful launching effect of one, preferably two, glasses of water. The same applies after a loaded dinner in or out of the home; charge the system with a tall glass of water as early as possible after the meal. Wonders never cease.

MANAGE YOUR GUT "EXIT" ACTIVITY

Problems relating to digesting, absorbing, and eliminating food can cause waste-product accumulation within the body. Inadequate excretion of human waste can be a meaningful contributor to the condition known as leaky gut.

While a daily poo is standard for most people, two or three times a day, or as often as you eat a meal, can be better (Gerasimo, 2017). What is passed through your fecal matter is just as important as what is eaten.

EATING OUT: MANAGE YOUR EATING HABITS

Eating out can often mean an extra 200 or more calories per day; also, a greater tendency to consume less nutritious food, in particular, a lesser consumption of plant foods.

Fast food restaurants are almost a curse on a core desire to manage weight; there is a greater risk of becoming overweight or obese. The preponderance of meat dairy, fat, and sugar in fast-food fare means high calorie-dense food consumption coupled with the transfer content of available dishes. Combined with bread and exposure to white flour in various forms, the overall low-fibre content spells negative health effects.

Gluten

Problems relating to gluten intolerance are discussed in Chapter 8. Individuals who suffer from gluten intolerance need to be alert to the avoidance of food items which contain gluten. The list of traditional foods, including restaurant prepared items, is quite lengthy. Some restaurants do offer gluten-free meals.

An extensive listing, indicated hereunder, provides considerable information on what an individual should be alert for in and out of the home with respect to the avoidance of gluten-containing foods:

1. Eggs served at restaurants; pancake batter is sometimes put in scrambled eggs and omelets
2. Cheesecake
3. Tofu is gluten free—but! be careful when fried
4. Meat substitutes may be made with seitan (wheat gluten); e.g. vegetarian burgers and sausage, imitation seafood, or bacon
5. Salad dressings may contain malt vinegar, soy sauce, flour
6. Cream-based soups; flour may be used as a thickener or may contain barley
7. Tortilla and tortilla chips: check if entirely corn-based

8. Potato chips: the seasonings may contain malt vinegar or wheat starch
9. French fries: the batter may contain wheat flour
10. Energy bars: may contain wheat and non-gluten-free oats
11. Sauces and gravies: many uses wheat flour as a thickener
12. Avoid traditional soy sauce; opt for tamari
13. Pastas, ravioli, dumplings, and couscous
14. Noodles, chow mein, egg noodles (rice and mung bean noodles are an exception)
15. Breads, crackers, pretzels, and pastries, including croissants, pita, naan, bagels, muffins, donuts, and rolls
16. Baked goods: cakes, cookies, pie crusts, brownies
17. Breakfast foods: pancakes, waffles, French toast, crepes, biscuits
18. Stuffing, dressings, croutons
19. Malt beverages, beer
20. Distilled alcoholic beverages and vinegars (most are gluten-free)

WEIGHING ONESELF: TRACKING PERSONAL PROGRESS

Regular weight checks are considered vital for achieving progress in weight management. Recommendations vary; however, at least once a day. If once a day, one recommendation is on mornings before breakfast. Twice a day is supposedly more effective; first thing in the morning and last thing at night.

CONTROLLING BLOOD SUGAR LEVELS

Some level of consciousness is necessary with respect to the relationship between blood sugar levels and fat deposit on the body. Food item selection and patterns of consumption are very relevant in the management of obesity.

Splitting the Meal: Reduce the Quantity Eaten at Any One Time

Eat five to six times a day and spread them out somewhat evenly. This helps to keep metabolism high, provides a feeling of fullness, minimizes binging, and assists in controlling blood sugar (glucose) spiking.

THE MICROBIOME: GUT BACTERIA

In a more general sense, your personal microbiome would seem to have a wholistic relevance to your general good health. An interesting kind of summary statement: The health of your entire bacterial community—your personal microbiome—is supposedly one of the great predictors of a long and happy life.

Remember that the quality of your gut bacteria may well be an important source of the difficulty you encounter in weight management.

A damaged gut can mean leaky gut; undigested food products cross into the blood stream and lead to inflammation in different parts of the body, including the brain and cardiovascular system. This chronic inflammation is associated with eight of the top 10 leading causes of death. Leaky gut is associated with difficult weight management. It can seriously limit achievement in weight control.

Processed foods and animal products are pro-inflammatory compared to the anti-inflammatory qualities of whole plant foods. The advice for successful weight management includes avoiding lectin and gluten-rich foods as a factor in the repairing of the gut lining, again, by eliminating processed and packaged foods.

The struggle with obesity demands serious consciousness of the nature of good and bad bacteria. If leaky gut is suspected or confirmed, the effort at repairing the gut lining requires that food consumption choices aim at fostering and maintaining good bacterial stock.

The core principle is to avoid, or at least reduce, food items which damage the gut, contribute to inflammation, or boost the presence of bad bacteria.

Some pointers on what foods to avoid to manage the microbiome:

1. Alcohol (increases inflammation, lowers immunity level, feeds bad bacteria)
2. Artificial sweeteners
3. Dairy (milk, cheese, yogurt, butter)
4. Foods containing gluten
5. Processed foods
6. Excessively starchy foods (wheat flour, potatoes, rice, corn)
7. Saturated fats (reduce or avoid butter, cheese, cream, coconut oil)
8. Sugar

Probiotics are important in the health of the digestive system, a significant factor in the promotion of a healthy immune system. Regular addition of probiotics to the diet facilitates maintenance of a healthy ratio of good bacteria. Good digestive health is a critical input in the battle against obesity.

Sit while you eat and eat less. Individuals eat five times more when in a rush and standing. Sitting facilitates a greater consciousness of the eating function; fullness is more readily recognised.

FOOD LABELLING

Food labelling is intended to be based on scientific analysis and should aim at providing the consumer with basic, current information. It should help consumers make choices in the pursuit of good health. It is even more important if specific personal problems demand that selected food items be avoided at all costs.

Remember that nutrition labels are not always factual; keep in mind that errors, to a limited extent, are usually allowed by authorities responsible for "standards" control.

Be suspicious of labels which read low or reduced fat or fat-free; they all have added sugars. Beware of Olean (aka olestra), a carb used extensively in snack foods, such as potato chips and similar products.

Take note that sugar content is often hidden, such as under HFCS and fruit juice concentrates. Be aware of fruits high in sugars—that is, high and medium glycemic fruits. They raise sugars faster and higher and are to be eaten less frequently or avoided. Fruits with a glycemic index of 70 or more: very ripe bananas, pineapple (can vary with country of origin), and watermelon. Moderate glycemic index fruits (56–69) include cantaloupe, figs, grapes, kiwi, and lychee; eat in moderation.

Be cautious in arriving at conclusions relating to comparative quality and quantity calories.

SUMMARY

Keep in mind the many little things that contribute to your gaining or losing weight. The umbrella idea of a change in lifestyle is a constant reminder that there are no shortcuts and that the target of sustained, successful weight management in the struggle against obesity is not an overnight initiative.

This review publication covers the important basics; keep it handy.

References

"Burn Fat Like a Kid Again". Woman's World. July 27, 2020

"Heal your Guy, Lose your Belly Fat". First For Women Magazine. June 27, 2016

"I Fought Fatigue and Won". First For Women Magazine. April 16, 2012

"Naturally Savvy's Label Lessons in Tonic". Jan/Feb 2020

"Obesity Worldwide-Statistics and Facts". www.statistica.com

"Prenatal Stress Associated with Infant Gut Microbes". Infant Health, UP FRONT – New and Events. Chiropractic and Naturopathic DOCTOR. July/August 2021

"The Fundamentals of Strengthening Your Core". Experience Life, October 2017

The link between dehydration and metabolism. *Wellness Magazine.* https://www.ewellnessmag.com/article/the-link-between-dchydration-and-metabolism

"The Most Powerful, Effective Digestive Enzymes". Natural Factors.com

"The Obesity Epidemic. Breaking North America's Bank". Chiropractic and Naturopathic DOCTOR. January/February 2021

"The Role of Mental Health in Obesity Management". Adult Obesity Clinical Practice. The Canadian Association of Bariatrics, Physicians and Surgeons. Canada Adult Obesity Clinical Practice Guidelines. Internet November 2022

"Try Tabata". Fit Body Section. Experience Life; October 2017

"Turbo Diet Tea". Woman's World. 2019

"Why Isn't My Low Carb Diet Working?" For Women First Magazine. July 31, 2017

(2017, July 31). Your water bottle could be making you fat. *First for Women.*

Adult Obesity in England; Health Survey for England, (HSE), 2017 and 2018 Fact Sheet, Internet

Agaston, Arthur M.D. The South Beach Diet, Rodal 2003

Amanda MacMillan in "You asked: Can Eating Breakfast Help your Metabolism" in "Modern Diet Custom Answered". The Source of Weight Loss. Time, Special Edition 2019

Anderson, Rosemary. "Diet as Medicine". *Trek Magazine.* Fall/ Winter 2022

Antonia Zerbisias, "Wonder Weight Woman" Article in F. Section, Toronto Star, November 15, 2002

As cited from: Chemo Preventative Activities of Phytochemicals. International Journal of Molecular Science. 21(s), 2020. Special Issue, Beneficial Properties of Green Tea Catechins (Internet May 2020)

Austin, Denise. "Walk off 3x more Belly Fat". First For Women Magazine. April 16, 2012

Baker, Efuha. 15 Minute Calorie Burn Workout. Shek Wah Tong Printing Press Ltd., China 2010

Ballou, S., and Anthony Lembo, Prashant Singh, Vikram Rangan, Johanna Iturrino and Judy Nee. (2019, September 18). Study: obesity associated with abnormal bowel habits – not diet. https://www.bidmc. org/about-bidmc/news/2019/09/obesity-and-diarrhea#:~:text=After%20 controlling%20for%20dietary%2C%20physical,normal%20bowel%20 habits%20or%20constipation

Barnes,Zara."10 Fruits with Super High and Low Sugar Counts' in Sugar Detox Made Easy.2019

Baxter, Whitney. "Microbiome Balance (Importance of Gastrointestinal Health for Thyroid Hormone Conversion". Chiropractic + Naturopathic Doctor. May/June 2021 pp 10-11

Beil, L. (2011, Jan 11). Lights out. in *The Oprah Magazine.*

Biotrust, Commentary on the Keto Diet; Jan 9, 2020

Brix, Jennifer. "Probiotics & Fibre for Peak Mental Health. Women's Voice Magazine. Spring 2020

Bussin, James. "The Three Greatest Risk Factors to your Cardiac Health". Tonic. Jan-Feb, 2020

Calton, Mira and Jayson; in For Women First Magazine. July 31, 2017 (email: health@firstforwomen.com)

Cassie Irwin, "Optimizing the Gut – Brain – Heart Connection" (Get Riddance to Bad Gut Bacteria) in Healthy Directions. Autumn 2019

Cassity, J. (2012). 100 simple ways to lose weight. *Prevention.* https://www.prevention.com/weight-loss/ a20437039/100-easy-tricks-to-move-more-and-lose-weight/

Charney, Thalia. "Post Meal Indigestion" in Vista. No.127, Nov/Dec. 2019

Oaklander, Mandy. "Rx for Exercise". TIME, val 188; No 10-11, 2016

Colbert, Don, M.D., Let Food be your Medicine (Dietary Changes Proven to Prevent or Reverse Diseases). Worthy Press, 1987 / 7A. Colbert, Dr. Keto Zone Diet, Special Ministry Edition, Worthy Publishing, 2017 Colbert Don, MD .Let Food be Your Medicine: Dietary Changes Proven to Prevent or Reverse Diseases. Worthy Press.2016

Colbert, Don. Hormone Health Zone. SILOAM. 2019

Conrad, Miller. "Far Stronger Lungs, More, More" in The Epoch Times. December 1-7, 2022.

Conrad, Miller. "Far Stronger Lungs, More, More" in The Epoch Times. December 1-7, 2022.

Cox, Jennifer." Fitness and Virtual Reality CSA News, Summer 2023

Cruize, Jorge. "LA's Slim-Quick Secret: Tea Toxing" For Women First Magazine. July 31, 2017

David Katz and Joe Kila, "Clean up your Diet" in Sugar Detox Made Easy, 2019

Davies, Alisha and Bhatia Tazeem. "Can the NHS Help Tackle the UK's Obesity Epidemic". The Nuffield Trust, UK. Blog Post 20 March, 2015

Davis, W. (2011). *Wheat belly*. Penguin Random House.

Debra Goldstein, " How to Prepare for your Detox" in Sugar Detox Made Easy .2019 ..

DeSoto, L. (2022, April 30). Is breakfast really the most important meal of the day? *Medical News Today*. https://www.medicalnewstoday.com/articles/is-breakfast-really-the-most-important-meal-of-the-day

Denney, Amy. "Cultivating our Gut Microbes to Stiffle Disease".The Epoch Times, April 13-19, 2023.

Denney, Amy. "How the Gut Cures and Creates Disease. A Medical Frontier. The Epoch Times; April 20-26, 2023

Dr. Amy Lee, Internet video on Weight Management (nutific.com)

Dr. Oz's Best Slim Down Tips Ever. Dr. Oz Guide Prevention Special. 2020

Dr. Oz's Best Slim Down Tips Ever. Dr. Oz Guide Prevention Special. 2020

English, Tannya. "African American Women and the Obesity Epidemic Report." Kaiser Health News. December 2011

Elflein, John." Share of Adults Worldwide who were obese in 2020 and forecasts to 2035 by Gender". www.Statistica.com

F.A.O. "United Nations calls for urgent action to curb the rise in hunger and obesity in Latin America and the Caribbean". News; Santiago de Chile. November 12, 2019

Finlay, Brett and Finlay J. The Whole Body MICROBIOME.

Fitz-Ritson, Don. "Aging: Cognition and Exercise". Chiropractic and Naturopathic DOCTOR. March/April 2021

Food and Agriculture Organization (FAO) and The Caribbean Development Bank (CDB). A Study on the State of Agriculture in the Caribbean. 2019

Food Revolution Network. "70 Doctors Reveal Secrets to a Healthy Microbiome". Website: "The interconnected series.com". November 23, 2021

For Women First Magazine. July 31, 2017

Funk, Anna. 'Fire in the Belly: How Your Diet, Microbes and More Contribute to your Gut's Health". Discover Magazine. July-August 2020

G. Joe, "Burn Fat Safely While Boosting Your Mood, Memory and Metabolism Naturally" in a collection of writings on Sane Whey. Internet: Sane Solution.com

Gerasimo, Pilar. "Revolutionary Act #35: Move It Out" in Experience Life, October 2017

Gorman,R M."Solving the Sugar Puzzle"in What To Eat For Life., Special Eating Well Edition.2020

Gottfried, S. (2021, August 30). Ketogenic diet: who benefits and who is at risk? https://www.saragottfriedmd.com/ketogenic-diet-who-benefits-and-who-is-at-risk/

Greene, Bob. "Get Moving" in The Oprah Magazine, Oprah's Next Chapter; Vol 12 (1). January, 2011.

Greger, M. How Not to Diet. Flatiron Books. 2019

Greger, M. https://nutritionfacts.org/video/breakfast-like-a-king-lunch-like-a-prince-dinner-like-a-pauper/#:~:text=Since%20they%20were%20all%20eating,two%20inches%20off%20their%20waistline.)

Gundy, Stephen. Internet: https:.//gundrymdm.com May 2020

Hallie Levire, "The Definitive Guide to Body Fat in the Science of Weight Loss". Time, Special Edition p.34

Hanna, Joseph. "Keeping in Balance: Probiotics can help Offset the Side Effects of Antibiotics". Costco Connections, Sept/Oct. 2019

Harvard Health Publishing, Harvard Medical School "Should You Try the Keto Diet ?. August 31, 2020"

Harvard Medical School. Core Exercises; Special Health Report. 2020

Harvard Medical School. A Guide to Men's Health Fifty and Forward. Special Health Report. 2020

Harvard Medical School. Special Health Report. Guide to Men's Health Fifty and Forward.2020

Harvard University. "Sitting many hours per day linked to higher dementia risk" ; Week in Review, Health Beat, Harvard Publishing, Harvard Medical School. 2023.

https://www.harvardhealthonlinelearning.com/courses/lose-weight-and-keep-it-off

Hicklin, T. (2019). Bacteria enriched in marathon runners. https://www.nih.gov/news-events/nih-research-matters/bacteria-enriched-marathon-runners#:~:text=Researchers%20found%20that%20marathon%20runners,used%20to%20enhance%20exercise%20ability.

Hochwald, Lambeth." One Meal a Day" in The Complete Guide to Intermittent Fasting. Central Health. 2022

http: //pages.sanesolution.com/clean-way-landingina/#transcript, (jan,2020)" The top 10 benefits of adding clean whey to your smoothies and baked goods"

James, Manyika and Dobbs, Richard. The Obesity Crisis Essay. The Cairo Renewing Global Affairs. 2015

James, Mary, ND. " Is your liver causing you weight gain and fatigue?" https://www.womenshealthnetwork.com/detoxification/is-your-liver-causing-your-weight-gain-fatigue-and-acne/

Jensen, Karen. "Its Never Too Early to Talk Heart Health". Women's Voice. Spring 2020

Jensen, Karen. "Storage to Fat Burning" in Women's Voice Magazine. Vol. 19-C, Special Edition – Rejuvenate Your Life. 2023

Karst, Karlene. "The Blue Zones" in Women's Voice Magazine. Vol. 19-C, Special Edition – Rejuvenate Your Life. 2023

Kaye, Maria. "The Miracle of Insulin". University of Toronto Magazine; Mississauga – St. George/Scarborough). Autumn 2021.

Kaye, Maria. "The Miracle of Insulin". University of Toronto Magazine; Mississauga – St. George/Scarborough). Autumn 2021.

Kosti R I et. Al. "The epidemic of obesity in children and adolescents in the world".Cent Eur J.Public Health.Abstract, Review, Pub Med; Advaned User Guide, NIH[www. uncoveringrareobesity.com]

Liebman, H.L. Anatomy of Exercise for 50+. Firefly Books Ltd., 2020

Littlemore, Richard. COLONISED: The Human Microbiome. Trek, a Publication of Alumni UBC. Spring 2019

Littlemore, Richard."10 Billion Mouths to Feed"; UBC Magazine/ Alumni UBC,Fall/Winter, 2022

Lombardi, Lisa. "The Fun Way to Make Fitness Stick in the Power of Habits". Special Time Edition. 2018

Maher, Lucy. "Fasting for Longevity" in The Complete Guide to Intermittent Fasting. Centenial Books. Centenial Health 2022

Mark Ley, L and Grunewald J, "Healthful Essentials". Experience Life. October 2017

Maxbauer, Lisa. "5:2 FASTING TOTALLY RESET My Body in the COMPLETE GUIDE YO INTERMITTENT FASTING (Eat What you Love and Lose Weight). Centenial Books; Centennial Health 2022

McCallum, Selina. Feature Article on Sashagai Ruddock (Women, Power, Highlighting Real Beauty). Toronto Caribbean News. March 4, 2020

McMorris, Megan. "The 5:2 DIET PLAN in The Complete Guide to Intermittent Fasting (Eat What you Love and Lose Weight). Centenial Books. Centenial Health 2022

Melone, Linda. "Unexpected Things that Mess With Your Memory". TIME magazine, Special Edition. THE SCIENCE OF MEMORY. 2019

Milner, Conan. "The Whole Body Influence of your Meal Microbiome" in The Epoch Times, Mind and Body Section. December 29, 2022.

Miscellaneous Notes; research/comments [2023] related to fat cells, diabetes exercise]by selected scientists-Dr Buguera and Dr Shirisha Avadhanula [Cleveland Clinic, Ohio, USA. Also Dr Bruce Buchholz [Karolinska Inst., Sweden], Dr.Shingo Kajimura, , Boston, Ohio, MA, USA and others of UC, San Francisco.

Morell, Sally Falon. "Who was Dr. Weston Price and Why Did He Matter" in The Epoch Times. December 1-7, 2022.

Mosley, M and Spencer, M. The Fast Diet. Atria Books. 2013

Mwange, Chege and Dickson Amugsi, African Population and Health Research Centre (APHRC); originally published in The Conversation. Quartz Africa. 2018

Myers, Amy, "Listen to your Thyroid" in Experience Life. October 2017

Noom, "What Is Noom (and how can it help you lose weight)?" December 18, 2022/ last updated February 25, 2023. https://www.noom.com/blog/what-is-noom-how-does-noom-work/

Oakland, Mandy. "Rx for Exercise; How Physical Activity Fortifies the Brain and Body" . September 2016.

ONNIT. "MCT OIL: What are it's Benefits and How It Works". Source: Internet: April 4, 2020

Panoff, Lauren. "The Best Probiotics for Women in 2020". ONNIT Academy; Internet March 2020

Pedre, Vincent Dr. Source Internet video ; 27 March 2020

Peterson, S.D. et al. Pharmacotherapy for Obesity Management. Canada Adult Obesity Clinical Practice Guidelines. Internet November 14, 2022

Petty, Chris. "Diet and Dogma". TREK. UBC 40. 2016

Pope, Kate, "How Stress Makes Us Gain Weight". Time – The Science of Weight Loss, Special Edition (no date)

Public Health Agency of Canada. *Canadian Risk Factor Atlas (CRFA),* 2020 edition. Public Health Infobase: https://health-infobase.canada.ca/crfa/

Pritikin, Robert. The Pritkin Weight Loss Breakthrough. A Signet Book. Jan,1999

Ramdeo, J. (2023, June 14). Timothy's lifelong battle with obesity. *Trinidad and Tobago Guardian.* https://www.guardian.co.tt/news/timothys-lifelong-battle-with-obesity-6.2.1730446.60be378cbc

Ratnesar, Romesh." Against the Grain". Time, December 15, 1997

Readers' Digest Association. SWAP AND DROP DIET ; New Canadian No Diet Revolution. 2012

Reed, Alex. Keto Diet Statistics in 2023; Latest US Data https://bodyketosis.com/keto-diet-statistics/

Retelny, Shanti, V. "Pucker Up". Costco Connection; Jan-Feb 2020

Rheaume, Kate. "Exercise Snacks – Build Muscle and Increase Longevity" in Women's Voice Magazine. Vol. 19-C, Special Edition – Rejuvenate Your Life. 2023

Scheiner, Gary Dr. "Dealing with High Blood Sugars after Meals". (Internet, June 2020)

Scheiner G. (2011). Strike the spike II. Dealing with high blood glucose after meals. *Diabetes self-management, 28*(1), 29–37. https://pubmed.ncbi.nlm.nih.gov/21323071/

Schmidt, T. https://www.unsw.edu.au/newsroom/news/2022/08/don_t-fall-for-the-snake-oil-claims-of-structured-water--a-chemi

Schwanbeck, Klaus. Meyer&Meyer, 2018

Shah, Adarsh. "Exercise and Sleep – How are they connected" in Tonic; Nov-Dec 2022

OTAKE, Shin. www.maxiworks.com. 2024.

Stanton, John. Running (The Complete Guide to Building Your Running Program). Penguin, Canada. 2010

Take a Note (Research Finding). Trek, a Publication of Alumni UBC. Spring 2019

Tang, Priscilla: Foundations of Health: A Breath of Fresh Air in the Whole Family, Fall 2021

Teychenne, Megan and Miller, Clint from The Conversation (Internet), Deakin University, Australia (July 2020) "Health Check: in terms of exercise, is walking enough?" https://theconversation.com/health-check-in-terms-of-exercise-is-walking-enough-78604

TIME. "Train Your Brain". in the Science of Memory.Special Edtion. 2019

The University of British Columbia. UBC Alumni Magazine. Fall/Winter 2022

The Zoomer Guide, Your Health, 100 Years Strong. 2022

Thomas, Nashua. "Now Nothing can Stop Me" in First for Women. March 10, 2014.

Travers, Colleen, "But I'm Already on a diet I like" in The Complete Guide to Intermittent Fasting. Centenial Health, 2022.

University of Fyraskyla. "Physical Activityof Older People Requires Tailored Monitoring". University of Fyraskyla, Finland in News and Events; DOCTOR, Chiropractic + Naturopathic, July/August 2020

USA Today, https://tlccarlisle.com/

Vaccariello, Liz. The Digest Diet. Reader's Digest 2012

Vicki Shanta Retelny, "Picker Up: Try Apple Cider Vinegar. Costco Connections, Jan/Feb 2020

Vij, V. A., & Joshi, A. S. (2013). Effect of 'water induced thermogenesis' on body weight, body mass index and body composition of overweight subjects. *Journal of clinical and diagnostic research : JCDR, 7*(9), 1894–1896. https://doi.org/10.7860/JCDR/2013/5862.3344

Vysohlid, Michelle. "Optimal Health with Functional Nutrition". Vista Issue No. 127

WALSH, M.D. "Going the Distance" in The Complete Guide to Intermittent Fasting. Centenial Books; 2022

Wang, Youfa et al." The global childhood obesity epidemic and the association between socio-economic status and childhood obesity".Int Rev Psychiatry,Abstract. June 2012

WHAT TO EAT FOR LIFE. Special Eating Well Edition. (Principles to Eat and Live By). Updated Reissue. 2021

Wiliam David M.D., Wheat Belly. Harper Collins Publishers Ltd. 2011

Woman's World. Jan 13, 2021

Woman's World. Mar 13, 2023.

Women's Voice Magazine. Spring 2020

Women's World. Jan 25, 2021

Wyse, Tiffany. "Ask a Herbalist". In the Whole Family. Healthy Planet. Spring 2020

Yang, Jingduan. "Researched Benefits of Intermittent Fasting in Mind and Body Section of the Epoch Times. Jan 26 – Feb 1st, 2023.

Yee, Colleen, Sandman. "Bye-Bye Jiggly Fat" in First For Women Magazine. July 31, 2017

Additional Recommended Resources

1. John Hopkins University, Division of Endocrinology, Diabetes , , Department Nov 2020
2. www.onnit.com
3. www. ???.integrstivepro.com or www.??.wyldenaturalhealth.com
4. http//pubmet.ncbl.nim.gor/265485861/ - National Library of Medicine. National Centre for Biotechnological Information.27 March 2022
5. www.CDC Centre for Disease Prevention and Control. http/www. cdc.gov./obesity/data/adult – Adult Obesity Facts
6. Dirt to Dinner.com (global food, sustainable agriculture)
7. www.hsph.HarvardUnviversity
8. Website of Harvard University, Division of Endocrinology, Diabetes
9. www.dietdoctors.com/health/insulinresistance - what you need to know about insulin resistance
10. www.dietvsdisease.org
11. www.nccih.gov
12. www.nature.com
13. www.saragotfriedmd.org
14. www.webmd.com
15. www.health.harvardedu/stayinghealthy/shouldyoutrytheketodiet
16. WWW.HEALTH.HARVARD.EDU
17. https://obesitycanada.ca/understanding-obesity/
18. https://www.The Guardian.com: society.UK 2023
19. https://en.wikepedia.org/adipocytes#brown_fatcells. 2023